MW01031916

MILFORD, MI 48381

RECEIVED

APR 0 2 2018

UNDERSTANDING
FIBROMYALGIA

Also by Naheed Ali

Understanding Lung Cancer:
An Introduction for Patients and Caregivers

Understanding Celiac Disease:
An Introduction for Patients and Caregivers

Understanding Chronic Fatigue Syndrome:
An Introduction for Patients and Caregivers

Understanding Alzheimer's:
An Introduction for Patients and Caregivers

Understanding Parkinson's Disease:
An Introduction for Patients and Caregivers

Arthritis and You:
A Comprehensive Digest for Patients and Caregivers

Diabetes and You:
A Comprehensive, Holistic Approach

The Obesity Reality:
A Comprehensive Approach to a Growing Problem

UNDERSTANDING FIBROMYALGIA

An Introduction for Patients and Caregivers

Naheed Ali

ROWMAN & LITTLEFIELD
Lanham • Boulder • New York • London

Published by Rowman & Littlefield
A wholly owned subsidiary of The Rowman & Littlefield Publishing Group, Inc.
4501 Forbes Boulevard, Suite 200, Lanham, Maryland 20706
www.rowman.com

Unit A, Whitacre Mews, 26-34 Stannary Street, London SE11 4AB

Copyright © 2016 by Rowman & Littlefield

All rights reserved. No part of this book may be reproduced in any form or by any electronic or mechanical means, including information storage and retrieval systems, without written permission from the publisher, except by a reviewer who may quote passages in a review.

British Library Cataloguing in Publication Information Available

Library of Congress Cataloging-in-Publication Data

Names: Ali, Naheed, 1981– , author.
Title: Understanding fibromyalgia : an introduction for patients and caregivers / Naheed Ali.
Description: Lanham : Rowman & Littlefield, [2016] | Includes bibliographical references and index.
Identifiers: LCCN 2015041832 | ISBN 9781442226593 (cloth : alk. paper)
Subjects: | MESH: Fibromyalgia.
Classification: LCC RC927.3 | NLM WE 544 | DDC 616.7/42—dc23 LC record available at http://lccn.loc.gov/2015041832

♾ ™ The paper used in this publication meets the minimum requirements of American National Standard for Information Sciences Permanence of Paper for Printed Library Materials, ANSI/NISO Z39.48-1992.

Printed in the United States of America

Understanding Fibromyalgia is dedicated to my readers, to fibromyalgia sufferers, and to all who provided encouragement and support for my research.

This book represents reference material only. It is not intended as a medical manual, and the data presented here are meant to assist the reader in making informed choices regarding wellness. This book is not a replacement for treatment(s) that the reader's personal physician may have suggested. If the reader believes he or she is experiencing a medical issue, professional medical help is recommended. Mention of particular products, companies, or authorities in this book does not entail endorsement by the publisher or author.

CONTENTS

IV: IRON WILL TO FACE FIBROMYALGIA

AUTHOR'S NOTE

Understanding Fibromyalgia is not meant entirely for medical professionals, yet the nonmedical reader may encounter advanced medical terminology as disbursed throughout the writing. This is often necessary to keep the book in line with the intended comprehensive review of fibromyalgia, and because certain medical concepts necessitate clarification well beyond just a modest introduction. A glossary has been placed near the back of the book to explain complex lexicon to those who are not familiar with the language of medicine. Italicized words are further defined later on in the glossary.

PREFACE

Fibromyalgia is a condition that can surface as fatigue, muscle stiffness, and pain, affecting the patient's ability to conduct a normal life. It blights muscles, tissues, and joints, causing *chronic* pain, also called *myofascial* pain syndrome or *fibromyositis*. The pain sweeps through the body, leading to discomfort and distressing tendons, ligaments, and skeletal muscles. Fibromyalgia (FM) also induces pain in the tender points of the body. The number of tender points that can be active at any one time may vary over time and can be impelled by certain circumstances, such as stress. The person suffers aches in the shoulders, lower back, neck, knees, waist, and buttocks. In its development, FM moves throughout several regions. Moreover, the pain is due to biological problems in the brain.[1]

Tender points are not large areas of pain, nor are they extents that are characterized by deep pain. They are more like superficial areas or points that can exist anywhere on the person from the back of the neck to the knees. The tender points can be identified by the fact that they are normally more sensitive than the adjoining areas and are considered a classic sign of FM.[2]

DIFFICULTIES IN RECOGNIZING THE NATURE OF PAIN IN FIBROMYALGIA

In many cases, it is difficult to recognize pain as FM because symptoms are similar to other diseases. Disease confirmation can take a long time (up to five years in some cases) and is based on the patient's symptoms and a diagnosis of exclusion, requiring careful attention. No single test can detect FM. Laboratory testing is not required for diagnosis, but it can help evaluate the symptoms. The doctor will order tests to gage the *erythrocyte sedimentation rate* (ESR or "sed rate"), the C-reactive protein (CRP) levels, and thyroid function, and will order a complete blood count and a metabolic panel. He will also conduct a physical examination to identify other disorders that might also be present.[3]

In 1990, the multicenter criteria committee of the American College of Rheumatology elaborated the most accepted classification criteria for the study of FM. The "ACR 1990" defines FM according to the presentation of a history of persistent widespread pain, lasting more than three months and affecting all four quadrants of the body; at least eleven of the eighteen tender points must be involved. The ACR criteria for patient classification were settled primarily as inclusion criteria for research and were not intended as a medical diagnosis. The criteria have since morphed into the diagnostic benchmarks accepted by physicians. The American College of Rheumatology classification criteria is now used in standard FM diagnoses.[4]

Many who suffer from FM are currently undiagnosed. Between 80 and 90 percent of FM patients are women, but it can affect anyone. The diagnosis is essential to propitiously managing care leading to a healthier life. Chronic pain, fatigue, and sleep problems are symptoms that can lead to a diagnosis, while depression and anxiety are also symptoms of FM. Many indicators may become chronic if the patient does not seek restorative treatment.[5]

FIBROMYALGIA AND QUALITY OF LIFE

A person affected with FM can experience a significant decrease in quality of life. The sometimes unbearable pain can lead to a change in routine, impacting both work and social life, and so treatment is important. Because it is difficult to live a full life while suffering widespread pain, the origins of the pain must be ascertained properly and treated accordingly. The problem is in the brain, but it affects the entire body, from head to toe. The light at the end of the tunnel is that there are valuable medications to control the disease, and FM patients and caregivers can learn how to make certain lifestyle modifications.[6]

IMPORTANCE OF READING ABOUT FIBROMYALGIA

A neurological disease is a condition that impacts the brain, spine, and nervous system. There are hundreds of disorders that fall into this group, including FM. It is important to be aware of how these diseases can impact daily life. Diseases such as FM cause significant alterations in health. Education is one of the most powerful tools available. The importance of reading about health and neurological maladies such as FM may not be something most people would think to do when focused on disorders such as blood pressure, weight, or any of a variety of other conditions. Nonetheless, it is important for patients and caregivers alike to realize that these factors offer only a basic paragon of how healthy a patient may be at any point.[7]

Once FM sufferers begin to expand their knowledge of the body as well as the vast number of conditions and symptoms that can have a dramatic impact on the way they look and feel, they should begin to monitor their health for risk factors for various neurological impairments. Reading about FM specifically can funnel a patient's health by way of boosting awareness and allow the patient to make decisions that could dramatically improve the patient's quality of life. As the FM sufferer realizes the importance of scanning through information banks about health and neurological diseases, she will be much more likely to be proactive about decisions that influence health.[8]

I

Lead In

I

HISTORY OF FIBROMYALGIA

Fibromyalgia holds Latin and Greek roots: *fibro* essentially means "fibrous tissue"; *myos*, from Greek, means "muscles"; and *algos*, from Greek, means "pain."[1]

Fibromyalgia (FM) is not a new disease. It has existed for centuries. Hippocrates used the term *rheumatismos* for the first time in 400 BC as a description of pain. About AD 200, Galen, a Greek physician, wrote about widespread pain and called it *rheuma*. In the sixteenth century, FM was termed muscular *rheumatism*, with distinction between articular rheumatism with deformation and painful but not tissue-deforming musculoskeletal disorders.[2]

The religious figure Job may have been the first recorded case of FM. He was described as having "months of pain, day and night." This may be the primordial description of a fibromyalgia-like condition.[3]

Pain as a whole has been studied since the sixteenth century. Guillaume de Baillou analyzed muscular pain and rheumatic fever in 1592. Since the 1800s, British, German, and Scandinavian physicians wrote about rheumatism. In the eighteenth century, muscular rheumatism was studied, and in the nineteenth century many textbooks about muscular rheumatism were published. William Balfour, a physician from Edinburgh, described nodules in 1815 and came to the conclusion that nodules and pain were caused by *inflammation* in muscle connective tissue. He was the first to report on focal tenderness (tender points) in 1824. Charles Scudamore identified rheumatism with inflammatory action in 1827, confirming the idea of inflammation in fibrous tissues.

Francois Valleix established the trigger point concept, describing painful points in various body parts, proposing muscular rheumatism as neuralgia. In 1850, Johan Mezger, a Dutch physician, introduced massage to patient treatment, addressing the bands in muscles.[4]

In 1880, American physician George Beard referred to widespread pain by using the term *neurasthenia* and *myasthenia*. Daily stress was cited as the cause of pain, fatigue, and psychological disturbance.[5]

In 1904, William Gowers, a British neurologist, used the term *fibrositis* for the first time. Fibrositis showed a similarity to cellulitis, and Gowers viewed it first as lumbago and muscular rheumatism and second as a form of inflammation or swelling of the tissues. Gowers stated that the symptoms for the disease were immediate pain and asymptomatic sensitivity to mechanical compression, fatigue, and sleep problems that worsen with cold and muscular strain. Fibrositis was the accepted label for many decades until physicians discovered that many individuals did not have swelling.[6]

In 1913, Jones Llewellyn and Bassett Jones classified fibrositis as a disorder of articulation, bursa-like, neurologic, muscular, with the presence of gout, infectious, due to trauma, and rheumatism. In the 1950s fibrositis was designated as a myofascial pain syndrome, also known as fibromyalgia syndrome or FMS. For Charles Slocumb, fibrositis was the most frequent type of rheumatism. Janet Travell and Seymour Rinzler generalized the terms *myofascial trigger points* and *myofascial pain syndromes*.[7]

During World War II, sweeping occurrences of rheumatism were observed among British soldiers, which was attributed to stress and depression due to the living conditions they suffered in battle camp. Rheumatism was also reported among American soldiers. Edward Boland and William Corr called this *psychogenic rheumatism*.[8]

In 1937, James Halliday stated that muscular rheumatism was a form of a chronic psychoneurotic condition. He rejected the term *fibrositis* and preferred *psychogenic rheumatism*, a syndrome designating pain, stiffness, and soreness (which continues to be espoused today).[9]

In 1942, Thomas Graham described the neurological pain as fire—burning, sticking, biting, strongly aching, and rather irksome. In 1949, Graham wrote a chapter about FM in the book *Arthritis and Allied Conditions*, which made a relevant contribution for new discoveries and research.[10]

In 1968, Eugene Traut made a significant contribution to the concept of fibrositis still heard today. He observed pain in women (generalized ache, stiffness, fatigue, headache, colon inflammation, and poor sleep) and demonstrated the common tender points locations, affirming that women have more symptom locations and more tender points than men. [11]

The modern concept of FMS was arguably developed by Hugh Smythe, who was the first to describe the disease as a widespread pain syndrome, tiredness, poor sleep, stiffness, worsening and relieving factors, emotional disorders, and many tender points. Many of his concepts are used in the American College of Rheumatology (ACR) standards of 1990. He included sleep as a cause of the disorder. Harvey Moldofsky corroborated the concept, and came to the conclusion that serotonin deficiency causes sleep anomalies in FM sufferers. [12]

In 1981, Muhammad Yunus of the University of Illinois confirmed that pain, tiredness, and poor sleep conditions occur more commonly in FM patients. Fibromyalgia began to be considered a syndrome, validating that there are more tender points in FM patients. He added tissue swelling, paresthesia, headaches, migraines, and irritable bowel syndrome (IBS) to the budding list of symptoms. [13]

In 1989, James Hudson and Harrison Pope corroborated the interconnection of medical functional syndromes and many psychiatric disorders (depressive condition, panic, bulimia, and obsessive-compulsive distress), including depression in the symptoms of FMS. [14]

In 1999, Robert Bennett confirmed central sensitization in FMS, which was reviewed by Yunus in 2000, and he introduced the idea of central sensitivity disorders, including myofascial pain syndrome, jaw pain disorder, tension-type headaches, migraines, and chronic fatigue syndrome (CFS). Bennett used the term *central sensitivity syndromes* and later added sensitivity to chemical products (perfume, for example), post-traumatic stress illness, and depression as symptoms. [15]

In 1984, Frederick Wolfe identified the association of FM with many connective tissue diseases, for example, lupus and arthritis. [16] By 1991, Carol Buckhardt developed the Fibromyalgia Impact Questionnaire, which became widely used in studies and in treatment. [17] Gerald Granges and Geoffrey Littlejohn presented the evidence of clinical signs in FM in 1993. [18]

Since 1989, studies have shown associations between FM and genetic aggregations, showing an important significant connection with the HLA gene.[19]

A few important improvements have been made for the treatment of FM. Trials were conducted with amitriptyline, cyclobenzaprine, and tramadol. Physical exercise was recommended, but the impact of behavioral therapy was not decided.[20]

Fibromyalgia was once thought to be a mental disorder, but now, after many years of research, physicians know more about its nature. In the twentieth century, FM has begun to be perceived as a "real" disease. Technology has advanced and now sheds more light on the *diagnosis* and treatment of FM. As more and more information becomes available through scientific revelations and research, the face of FM is vacillating. The move to a better comprehension of the disorder is still slow but constant. Many physicians are dedicating themselves to study and treatment.[21]

The term *FM* came into generalized use in 1987, when the American Medical Association (AMA) recognized it as a disease for the first time. The term was designated in that same year by Goldenburg, in an article of the *Journal of the American Medical Association* (JAMA), explaining that the term *fibrositis* was inaccurate since many FM patients do not suffer from inflammation.[22]

CELEBRITIES WITH FIBROMYALGIA

Fibromyalgia can affect anyone, rich or poor, average person or celebrity. There are several artists who suffer from FM. The most noteworthy are as follows[23]:

Actor Morgan Freeman, Golden Globe winner for his role in *Driving Miss Daisy* and recognized for his astounding voice, began suffering the symptoms of FM after a car accident in 2008. Freeman has said he suffers significant pain, but he doesn't let that dissuade him from working and continues to perform his roles in film. Despite his chronic illness, he continues to be brilliant, intelligent, and likable. A large FM organization invited Freeman to become its spokesperson.[24]

Sinead O'Connor, the Irish Grammy winner and successful and controversial rock singer, also suffers from FM. She stepped out of the spotlight in 2003 owing to severe pain and fatigue, but her disease is now under control. Fibromyalgia does not prevent O'Connor from being an excellent singer. She has said that although FM has no cure, she has been able to manage her symptoms.[25]

Susan Flannery, a four-time Emmy Award–winning actress, was forced to cease working in 2007, but the star of *The Bold and the Beautiful* was able to later return to her role once her symptoms were under control.[26]

Michael James Hastings, Captain Mike of *The West Wing*, left his career after he began suffering from FM at the age of thirty. He has since become a national spokesperson for FM patients. He promotes *enzymatic therapy* to lull the disease.[27]

Rosie Hamlin, a prominent singer, retired from her musical career because of FM, and today she is a spokesperson for those who suffer from it. In 2004, Hamlin appeared on the cover of *Fibromyalgia AWARE*. She suffers memory loss, depression, burning sensations, *irritable bowel syndrome*, and pain. To get relief from these symptoms, she uses massage and acupuncture treatments, water exercises, and a diet and vitamin regimen.[28]

Janeane Garofalo, the hilarious comedienne and actress, suffers from FM. Garofalo looks to an antidepressant to combat the pain, and the result has been positive. She continues to make people laugh, and despite her disease she can smile and laugh too.[29]

Frances Winfield Bremer, wife of U.S. Ambassador L. Paul Bremer III, has suffered from FM symptoms for more than three decades. Although she suffers from terrible pain and fatigue, she continues to encourage other FM patients to cope with this painful disease. She appeared on the cover of *Fibromyalgia AWARE* to promote awareness of the disease and to encourage other patients who continue to cope with the illness. She and her husband are active members of and raise money for FM organizations.[30]

A. J. Langer, wife of an English earl, does almost everything she used to do before being diagnosed with FM. Her dream life was affected but not wholly damaged by FM.[31]

Florence Nightingale was one of the first well-known people to report she was afflicted with FM. In the nineteenth century she was a nurse in the Red Cross and the English army. She first exhibited symptoms of FM during her work in the Crimean War from 1854 to 1856.

Nightingale struggled with FM for many years. In 1896 she became bedridden, and she died in 1910 at the age of ninety.[32]

Mary McDonough, known for her role in *The Waltons*, suffers from FM. She also has *lupus* and *Sjögren's syndrome*. McDonough is an active spokesperson for lupus and FM organizations.[33]

Jo Quest used to be a glamour model and media figure who, in 1997, was diagnosed with FM, which she said has ruined her career.[34]

This disease does not discriminate between the rich or poor, the famous or the common folk. Many celebrities affected with this disorder have affirmed that most patients can find relief and manage a normal (or almost ordinary) life.[35]

2

CONNECTIONS BETWEEN FIBROMYALGIA AND CHRONIC FATIGUE SYNDROME

Do FM patients tire easily? Do chronic fatigue syndrome (CFS) patients also experience FM? Is there a scientific or a theoretical link between FM and CFS? The answer to all of these questions, often asked by FM patients, is yes. Fibromyalgia patients tire easily, often have lassitude, and are usually also diagnosed with CFS.[1]

In the end, FM and CFS are separate but related disorders. Many physicians consider FM and CFS to be manifestations of the same disease, and an individual can suffer from both. Some of the shared symptoms include the following[2]:

- reduced heart rate variability
- low blood pressure
- reduced aerobic capacity
- reduced brain blood flow
- increased *neuropeptide y*
- reduced salivary awakening to cortisol
- increased *IL-6*
- widespread pain
- fatigue
- poor or restless sleep
- constipation and *irritable bowel syndrome*
- chronic headaches or migraines

- *temporomandibular joint syndrome* (TMJ)
- cognitive or memory damage and difficulty concentrating
- dizziness
- worsened coordination
- allergies and asthma
- breastfeeding difficulties
- chemical sensitivities
- cold extremities (Raynaud's syndrome)
- dry or itchy skin (eczema)
- thinning hair
- husky voice
- infertility or miscarriages and menstrual irregularities
- muscle cramps
- puffiness around the eyes
- rashes
- decreased *libido*
- sluggishness
- tingling in extremities
- weight gain and difficulty losing weight

FM and CFS patients are more likely to also experience:

- fever
- swollen glands
- sore throat
- recurring yeast infections
- dry mouth (associated with *Sjögren's syndrome* and *hypothyroidism*)
- increased risk for cavities

These medical conditions can increase the usual symptoms of FM and CFS. Infections must be diagnosed early and treated to prune their impact on FM and CFS symptoms. The symptoms and abnormalities in both diseases can be documented in SPECT and PET scans, and it has not yet been determined whether the abnormalities are the origin or result of the disorders. Other similarities of FM and CFS include genetic factors (family members may also develop the diseases); environmental factors (physical trauma, infections, other acute and chronic diseases), especially with genetic predisposition; both disorders are rare;

the symptoms appear and disappear abruptly; symptoms are influenced by exercise; and neither disease has a cure. In both cases, psychiatric disorders also often transpire (30 to 60 percent of FM and CFS patients have some form of psychopathology, the most common being anxiety and depression). Both diseases are difficult to diagnose, but it is recommended that a doctor be consulted early so an inveterate diagnosis can be made and treatment can begin.[3]

Chronic fatigue syndrome is described as unexplained fatigue that is present for more than six months and negatively impacts daily activity; fatigue that does not disappear with rest; fatigue accompanied by muscle and joint pain, sore throat, tender lymph nodes, cognitive dysfunction, and sleep disturbance; and discomfort after physical exercise that persists for more than twenty-four hours. Chronic fatigue syndrome is relentless; it does not go away. The most common symptoms are headache, tender lymph nodes, and weakness. Although the symptoms are similar to the flu, in CFS the symptoms are constant and continuous. Research shows that CFS sufferers have a lack of carnitine and acetyl-carnitine (a factor in energy metabolism). The supplement L-carnitine can recuperate health for CFS patients.[4]

Fibromyalgia presents more often in women as a result of psychological, biological, and social influences. These diseases rarely affect men, but they are not excluded. Fibromyalgia and CFS primarily affect women between the ages of forty and fifty, although either disease can start in young adulthood. They can also develop in children. In the United States, about one hundred thousand people are afflicted with FM, and it is more common than CFS. Between 10 and 20 percent of the population suffer from fatigue. There are three echelons of severity in both FM and CFS[5]:

- mild cases—the patient can perform light tasks, but with difficulty
- moderate cases—decreased mobility and restriction in daily life activities
- severe cases—inability to perform any tasks at all

For both diseases, education, pharmacotherapy, *cognitive behavioral therapy*, and exercise are recommended. The patient must be aware that FM and CFS are chronic conditions, although they are not progressive and do not cause inflammation. Medications most often prescribed for both diseases include antidepressants, antianxiety medications, and *analgesics*. Low doses of naltrexone (LDN) is a great elixir to alleviate the pain. A patient's mental health must be improved through behavioral changes. Additionally, adequate sleep level can alleviate the most common symptoms. Patients are advised to sleep seven to nine hours daily, preferably at night.[6]

Excessive exercise causes fatigue, sleep disturbance, distress, and pain, but for patients with CFS even minimum exercise can cause these persistent symptoms. Studies show FM and CFS patients exercise less than nonpatients; often they are less active because of anxiety. Due to inactivity, FM and CFS patients are 20 to 30 percent weaker than nonpatients. Aerobic training programs are recommended to improve fitness, diminish fatigue and pain, diminish heart rate and the rate of perceived exertion, increase functional capacity, and diminish symptoms. Light aerobic exercises for thirty minutes per day, such as walking and cycling, can be done as long as symptoms are not present as mentioned above. Aquatic aerobics can also ease pain, but the water temperature must be adequate. Stretching exercises, performed at home or in the gym, are beneficial in the treatment of FM and CFS, but they can be dangerous if the exercises are not performed correctly. Guidelines must be followed to prevent injury through stretching: warm up the muscles before stretching, make slow movements, and control breathing. Workouts must be performed at a comfortable room temperature.[7]

WHAT IS THE IMPACT OF THE CONNECTION BETWEEN FM AND CFS ON PATIENTS?

Fibromyalgia and CFS affect the patient's life dramatically. Pain and fatigue are a barrier to managing a normal life. The patients must change their habits to continue living copiously and look for help with confronting both diseases. A patient's social life is often impacted.[8]

Chronic fatigue syndrome, like FM, is a complex and serious condition. Between 20 and 70 percent of FM patients meet the criteria for CFS. The diagnosis of CFS is performed through clinical examination as well as laboratory testing. People with CFS are susceptible to developing FM as well as other illnesses such as obesity, insulin resistance, metabolic syndrome, irritable bowel syndrome, depression, and chemical sensitivity. Many of these disorders also betide in FM patients. The FM and CFS patient must undergo medical treatment, but achieving a good result is as complex as the disease. There is no cure for either disorder, and symptom variation occurs constantly. The patient must enter a health program to get relief from the symptoms these disorders cause. The patient must consider both FM and CFS as well as other diseases that may be presenting at the same time. The most annoying and cumbersome symptoms must be diagnosed and treated, using drug therapy to manage the symptoms. People with CFS and/or FM should learn to cope with both diseases.[9]

For drug therapies, it is recommended to use as few drugs as possible because of the side effects these medications can cause. The treatment should begin with small doses, snowballing until reaching the optimal dose. The use of narcotics is contraindicated for the relief of pain. It is recommended that CFS patients use acetaminophen, aspirin, or nonsteroidal medicines. Sleep medications are not recommended for CFS patients. The symptoms of depression must be treated with antidepressants. An adequate diet should be prescribed and followed. Comfrey, ephedra, kava, germander, chaparral, bitter orange, licorice root, and other herbal remedies must be avoided as part of treatment because they can trigger symptoms. Products such as milk, eggs, soy, wheat, and corn must be eliminated because they can trigger food allergies or intolerances.[10]

The patient should also consider nondrug therapies such as acupuncture, massage, deep breathing, relaxation techniques, yoga, or tai chi for the relief of pain. Before going to sleep, light exercise is recommended; activities such as puzzle games, crossword puzzles, and card games can be relaxing and are beneficial for memory improvement.[11]

The patient must seek treatment for symptoms such as anxiety, grief, depression, anger, and guilt that has virtually usurped his life. It is recommended that the patient seek support from organizations that work with FM and CFS patients. Fibromyalgia and CFS are so chronic that they can affect the entire family. The patient must learn how to have a meaningful life, avoiding the sensation of uselessness. In both diseases, the patient must learn to face the symptoms and the emotional problems that are often associated with them.[12]

Fibromyalgia and CFS can cause life changes throughout the course of the disease, such as a loss of independence, livelihood, and financial security. Patients of either may also see changes in their relationships with family, friends, and colleagues; daily life can be altered; and memory and concentration problems can affect the patient at work or at school. It is recommended that the patient seek support to overcome these issues as soon as they begin. To face these dramatic changes, the patient must look for aid, such as professional counseling (psychotherapy), to help overcome depression and anxiety; the sufferer should participate in support groups, which share counsel, tips, and experiences for facing both diseases. Individuals who cannot work must realize a favorable situation in which to achieve independence and life fulfillment.[13]

Cognitive behavioral therapy (CBT) has proven effective in leading the patient to a better quality of life and overall well-being. Research has shown that CBT is appropriate to deal with these disorders. With graded exercise therapy (GET), the patient starts with minimal exercises until drawing near to the ideal level to keep the symptoms at bay. Recommended activities are stretching, walking, biking, and anything else the patient can perform comfortably. Nonimpact and low-impact aerobics have been proven to be significantly beneficial for the treatment of both diseases.[14]

Irritable bowel syndrome (IBS) occurs frequently in both diseases, debilitating the body and sinking the quality of life. When IBS occurs with FM and CFS, there can be a serotonin imbalance. One disease can trigger the other, and FM and IBS are linked to stress. So, the patient can have other symptoms including nausea and vomiting, gas, bloating, and abdominal distention. To treat IBS, changes must be made to the patient's diet. The use of coconut oil is recommended as it increases energy levels. Lifestyle changes must take place: caffeine, alcohol, and smoking must be avoided. Moreover, vitamins and minerals are essential parts of diet treatment[15]:

- Vitamin E relieves pain, cramps, and is beneficial for sleep.
- Vitamin C increases immune functions.
- Vitamin D regulates immune functions.
- Magnesium increases natural killer cells.
- Inositol is beneficial for the immune system.

- Malic acid improves cell functions.
- Amino acids produce energy.
- Zinc helps boost the immune system.
- Selenium increases antibody production.
- Fructooligosaccharides improve digestion and regulate intestinal flora.
- Vitamin B improves energy levels (a lack of vitamin B worsens fatigue and mental fogginess and can lead to a devitalized immune system).

Fibromyalgia and CFS sufferers are sometimes left to cope with sleep difficulties. Professional help can lead the patient to an apt sleep level. Sleep therapy is recommended, and to improve rest, clients can limit light and noise and maintain a comfortable bed and room temperature. Relaxing activities, such as reading and listening to soft music before bedtime, are suggested. The patient must try to ignore the presence of the clock while attempting to sleep.[16]

The amendments to daily life caused by FM and CFS are dramatic. The patient has little to no energy, suffers from memory loss, stress, and sensitivity to light, sound, cold, or heat. There are ways to alleviate the symptoms; treatment does not heal, but it can diminish the symptoms. No medication is consistently effective for the treatment of both diseases simultaneously.[17]

In addition, both disorders create limitations in the patient's life, and practical and psychological adaptations must take place. The patient must accept the deviations these diseases bring and must make lifestyle changes. Furthermore, the help and understanding of all family members is extremely important for the life improvement of the patient. The symptoms of both diseases are unpredictable, and the patient never knows what to expect the next day. Flexibility is a solution strategy to cope with the unpredictability of FM and CFS. Activity levels can be reduced by as much as 85 percent due to pain and fatigue. The family must develop skills to face the disease positively, improving the patient's life quality. As a matter of fact, the role the family plays is very important to bring about improved sleep, consistent activity level, and stress control, as stress worsens the symptoms.[18]

Both disorders cause intense, hard-to-control emotions, which can intensify symptoms. Even sudden positive emotions can cause problems, causing a vicious cycle to take place: changes in emotions lead to symptom complications, which in turn lead to changes in emotions. It is recommended that the patient take a walk, rest, or listen to music in order to help discipline strong emotions.[19]

Stress occurs frequently—especially for long-term disorders. Fibromyalgia and CFS patients are more stress sensitive than nonsufferers. Although relationships may be marred, couples and family members must control stress to achieve a good life quality. The best way to control stress is with pacing. The patients must use care with scheduling so as to not be overwhelmed. For clients who work, changes may have to be made, such as changing from full to part time. Many want to continue working, but lack of energy is a significant problem. The work to be performed must not be overly demanding. Problems such as extra household tasks, financial strains, caregiving responsibilities, worries about the future, sadness, loss of companionship, and social obscurities must be taken in consideration and reduced when possible.[20]

Both diseases cause weather and sensory overload—changes in weather can interfere with a patient's health and severity of symptoms. Measures to avoid these symptoms ought to be made, such as going to public places in off-peak hours to bypass noise and other triggers.[21]

These disorders cause an economic impact of an average of $20,000 per person in lost wages ($180 billion annually) due to the incapacity to work. It affects the female workforce enormously. As money must also be splurged on the treatment and relief of the symptoms, the financial impact is increased.[22]

Both diseases have a psychological impact on a patient's life. FM and CFS affect the relationship in the family and social life in general. The patient and family must find ways to educate themselves on these conditions. Fibromyalgia and CFS can cause emotional damage for the patient and the family members and friends, oftentimes leading to feelings of fear, loneliness, isolation, anxiety, and panic. The FM and CFS patient develops a fear of rejection by others without reason. Therapy and counseling are advised for treatment of psychological effects. The patient must look for ways to manage the disease, and the help of family and friends is essential when struggling with functional and psychological issues that arise from these diseases. The patient must achieve emotional healing and be able to cope with this illness.[23]

For the family members and friends, it is heartrending to see the loved one consumed by pain and overwhelming fatigue. The family must understand the patient's condition and provide help and support. The family members must realize that the patient is not being lazy and does not exaggerate the effect of the symptoms. Fibromyalgia and CFS are considered real illnesses by countless physicians and must be regarded as chronic. The patient's difficulties ought to be acknowledged, and the entire family must cope with the fickleness of the disorder. There are many symptoms that are difficult to counter. Therefore, the family members must convince the patient that a medical condition is not a burden on them and life can continue to be conventional if the necessary measures are taken.[24]

Caregivers can teach the patient to learn about the gains from laughter—being in good spirits is instrumental in alleviating the symptoms. The patient must think positively and develop a good and appropriate attitude toward the condition. A healthy mind will contribute largely to diminishing the devastating effects FM and CFS can cause on social lives. Laughter is a healthy action that boosts the entire body, and desirable mental health is essential to coping with the disorder and bringing lasting health advantages. Simply put, first-rate humor makes life better. Protracted mental fitness will provide extended body health and will reduce the recurrence of the curt symptoms of FM and CFS. It is difficult to laugh or have good humor with pain and intense fatigue, but therapy can do wonders.[25]

WHAT ARE THE DIFFERENCES BETWEEN FM AND CFS?

The main difference between the two conditions is that in FM the predominant hindrance is pain, and in CFS the primary complaint is fatigue. Chronic fatigue syndrome occurs after a viral infection such as the flu, while FM is the result of a trauma (physical or emotional). Fibromyalgia has distinct pain sites (eighteen tender points), and these sites are not affected in CFS. In FM there is lack of inflammation, while CFS patients suffer from inflammation, including fever and swollen glands. There is a difference in sleep disturbances among patients with FM and CFS. There are other differences between the two diseases. Musculoskeletal pain occurs in FM but not in CFS; central sensitization is present in FM, in CFS it is only suggested. Immunological irregularities occur in CFS patients but not in FM sufferers. Patients of FM and CFS have different patterns of functional brain activity. In CFS, lower blood perfusion occurs in the brain stem, and in patients with FM there are lower levels of rCFB in the thalamus and caudate nucleus. Substance P is elevated in FM patients but not in CFS sufferers; RNaseL, a cellular antiviral enzyme, is normal in FM, but CFS patients have an elevated level. Furthermore, fibromyalgia symptoms can be relieved with heat and massage, but heat and massage therapy do not help CFS patients. IL-8 increases in FM and decreases in CFS. In FM there is a reduction of leptin levels, but leptin levels spike in CFS. The two diseases diverge in the central nervous system. Fibromyalgia does not cause joint pain, but CFS patients can suffer from it.[26]

Around the globe, FM researchers are mostly rheumatologists and nervous system experts, but immunologists and virus experts research CFS because FM is seen as a neurological disorder and CFS is marginally linked to viral infections. In FM, fatigue occurs with debilitating muscle pain; while CFS also involves pain, the most significant setback is a lack of energy.[27]

Other primary differences in the two diseases are: greater immune dysfunction in CFS and abnormal nerve response in FM; the HPA axis (the stress system) is stymied in CFS and the hypothalamus is affected in FM; the criteria for diagnosis of CFS include sore throat and lower-grade fever, but they are not considered in a FM diagnosis. Fibromyalgia is not progressive, but, in rare cases, CFS may become progressive; FM does not cause grave immune dysfunction, neurological symptoms, or intolerance to exercise; and CFS does not cause *allodynia*. A reduced level of BDNF (a nerve agent repair) is found in CFS. In FM the BDNF level is also abnormal, but it can be either higher or lower than normal.[28]

Symptomatically, research has shown an unambiguous link between FM and CFS, and hence, the patient must repress the symptoms in order to improve features of his life. Lifestyle changes must be implemented in both diseases, and with correct medication doses, symptoms can be significantly alleviated.[29]

3

HOW BODY SYSTEMS ARE AFFECTED SYMPTOMATICALLY BY FIBROMYALGIA

Symptoms and their occurrence may vary from person to person. They can cause problems in both work and social settings. Symptoms impact the central nervous system (CNS), the musculoskeletal system, the respiratory system, and the digestive system.[1]

Fibromyalgia is a medical condition of which one of the most common symptoms is pain. Depending on the source and nature of pain, and other types of symptoms, it can be treated by physicians aside from a neurologist. Some of the common symptoms of FM that must be addressed by physicians include the following[2]:

- pain
- headache
- fatigue
- anxiety
- depression
- urinary tract disorder symptoms
- memory and concentration problems
- morning stiffness
- sleeping disorder
- irritable bowel syndrome
- painful menstrual cramps
- tender points
- numbness in hands and feet

- tingling sensation in arms, hands, legs, and feet

FIBROMYALGIA AND THE CENTRAL NERVOUS SYSTEM

Common symptoms of FM are associated with pain. The pain experienced can be purely physical in nature, such as muscle pain, or psychological in nature, such as pain evoked by temperature or light. Researchers have suggested that overactive nerves in the CNS cause this pain. The CNS is made up of the spinal cord, the brain, and nerves, which helm a range of physical activities. The pain experienced in FM can be described as the following.[3]

- Tender point pain is experienced in any of the localized areas of the body. Patients diagnosed with tender point pain normally experience aches in multiple points on their body. The pain normally starts in or near the shoulder muscles and those of the neck. It gradually spreads from there to other areas of the body. The skin of such patients is highly sensitive, but they will not experience any pain in joints or any inflammation.
- Burning and aching pain comes with widespread stiffness and is often radiated from the fleck of origin to other nearby areas. When this happens, people are bound to experience constant pain, although the intensity may increase or decrease at different points. Most people suffering from the burning and aching pain find the experience mentally taxing and physically exhausting. This constant pain can vary in intensity according to the weather, the time of day or night, type of physical activity undertaken, stress, and inactivity. Research has indicated that disturbed sleep can intensify the pain as well.

There are several nervous system disorders that have symptoms closely associated with pain. One such disorder is known as *central pain syndrome*. It is a neurological condition that occurs in those people who have either suffered from or are suffering from multiple sclerosis, stroke, brain tumor, Parkinson's disease, limb amputations, spinal cord injury, or brain injury. People suffering from central pain syndrome experience a variety of pain sensations, with the most common sensation being the feeling of constant, burning pain. This emergent burning sensation can intensify even by the slightest touch. People suffering from this condition can also experience a loss of sensation in various areas of the body, especially the hands and feet.[4]

The first and foremost thing to understand here is that these pain symptoms are quite similar to those of FM. Secondly, tingling pain in hands or feet, localized pain in the neck and shoulders, and burning pain rising out of FM can further worsen the pain and sensitivity in people suffering from central pain syndrome. This is one of the many reasons why it is important to ward off FM through primary or secondary prevention methods.[5]

NERVOUS SYSTEM SYMPTOMS OF FIBROMYALGIA

Memory problems, with or without fibro fog, are as itemized[6]:

- difficulty following directions and making decisions
- difficulty paying attention
- difficulty recognizing faces and places
- difficulty remembering names of people and objects
- difficulty speaking known words
- distraction while executing a task
- long- and short-term memory difficulty due to chronic pain and sleep disturbance
- difficulty remembering routine activities
- blackouts and mental distraction because of difficulty concentrating
- disorientation when driving due to memory loss and difficulty concentrating
- difficulty distinguishing between colors because of impaired perception
- staring off into space trying to convoke thoughts because of feelings of disorientation
- forgetfulness
- dyscalculia (difficulty with math and numbers)

Dysphasia (speech problems) involves[7]:

- difficulty forming sentences and articulating words
- slowed or slurred speech, mainly in women (94 percent of female patients) and more common after the age of fifty
- difficulty following a conversation
- stammering or stuttering
- transposition of numbers or words when speaking or writing

Chagrins with motor skills include[8]:

- clumsy walking—the patient bumps into things and is off balance, and this can lead to the patient becoming disoriented
- difficulty holding or manipulating objects, which can hinder household chores, schoolwork, and manual labor tasks, and can cause the patient to frequently drop items because of coordination difficulty or muscle fatigue

Sensory overload aggravates the FM symptoms, and the sufferer can be subjected to temporary immobilization. The reasons for the sensitivities vary and are due to nervous system problems. The sufferer complains of irritability and overexcitement, leading to difficulty in performing daily activities. Some examples of sensory overload are[9]:

- noise intolerance that can lead to a crash and can cause immobilizing fatigue
- dysesthesia (numbness or tingling sensations) in hands and feet, possibly with swelling
- carpal tunnel syndrome, which can sometimes require surgery
- photophobia (sensitivity to sunlight, fluorescent, and incandescent light), which causes eye pain or discomfort leading to fatigue, anxiety, sweating, irritability, and sleep disturbances and can occur while reading or using the computer, driving at night, and watching TV
- increased sensitivity to odors, speed, and mixed sensory modalities
- chemical sensitivity (perfumes, cleaning supplies, and other chemicals)
- sensitivity to foods
- sensitivity to mold and to yeast (on the skin)

- sensitivity to humidity and temperature, which causes excessive sweating
- hypersensitivity to vibration

Symptoms of confusion are [10]:

- feeling spaced out (the sensation of being a zombie or a sleep-walker)
- lack of attention
- difficulties with multitasking because the patient is unable to pay attention to more than one thing at a time

Balance problems can occur with fibromyalgia. Pilates, tai chi, and yoga are great means for treating balance. Walking sticks or canes are beneficial to eliminate falls associated with balance problems. Vertigo (dizziness), neutrally mediated hypotension (NMH) (a drop in blood pressure that causes symptoms similar to vertigo), and vasovagal syncope (fainting) are examples of balance predicaments. Balancing issues can cause [11]:

- fainting or the sensation of fainting
- blurred vision
- pallor
- tremulousness
- a sense of imbalance and associated neck extension or rotation
- a sense that the room is spinning
- dizziness
- nausea
- vomiting
- *nystagmus*
- tinnitus

Sleep disturbances are common among FM patients, and can be chronic. Other symptoms are worsened by poor sleep. Sleep deficit is a very significant issue. Patients should eliminate tobacco, alcohol, and caffeine to help improve sleep. In FM patients, sleep disorders are related to the somatic symptoms, and sleep quality is associated with musculoskeletal tenderness, so less sleep means more active tender points. Sleep disorders must be treated because unrefreshing slumber can cause pain and fatigue. Although sleep can last between eight and ten hours, it is not always a restorative siesta in FM patients. Women suffer more with sleep reduction, and they often report oxygen saturation. Sleep apnea, which occurs more often in men, can cause headaches. The main sleep problems for both men and women include[12]:

- alertness late at night
- altered sleep
- *insomnia*
- excessive sleep
- fatigue
- *narcolepsy*
- unrefreshing (nonrestorative) sleep
- bad dreams or nightmares
- reversed diurnal sleep rhythms, which are not beneficial to good sleep quality level
- disrupted circadian rhythm
- *hypersomnia*, occuring in acute cases of FM
- morning tiredness
- *restless leg syndrome* (RLS), which may occur during sleep, causes an uncomfortable sensation in the legs causing the patient to move them constantly. Both FM and RLS have neurological causes. The interaction of medicines for both illnesses must be considered. RLS occurs ten times more often in FM patients.
- migraines, which can be alleviated with good sleep
- bruxism (teeth grinding)

Neurological problems are very frequent in FM; for example, hypertonic and hypotonic muscles, perceptual disturbances, and spatial instability.

MUSCULOSKELETAL SYMPTOMS OF FIBROMYALGIA

A person with fibromyalgia has difficulty holding objects because the cognitive sensation is very obstinate. A patient who has difficulty grasping a pen or pencil will also have difficulty manipulating objects. This symptom will impact the patient's ability to perform routine household chores, schoolwork, and manual labor tasks.[13]

Musculoskeletal (mechanical) pain is an omnipresent symptom of FM as the *myalgia* level is high in the muscles and tendons. The core symptom of FM is widespread pain. The pain is widespread and migratory due to the dysfunction of pain-processing areas of the CNS. The processing areas are linked with sodium channel and cellular ion transport dysregulation. The pain can be dull, sharp, shooting, severely aching, burning, or tingling. It is an ache that begins in the muscles and spreads, affecting many other body parts. The most common tender points are the neck, back, shoulders, legs, chest, inflamed rib cartilage, and head (presenting as a headache). Other pain symptoms include tender breasts, morning stiffness, muscle pain and spasms, twitching, muscle weakness, rib pain, restless leg syndrome, scalp pain, TMJ syndrome, and a voodoo doll sensation (pain sticking in various areas of the entire body). Excess or lack of exercise can render pain.[14]

The characteristics of FM-specific pain include[15]:

- *allodynia* (from touch); it is a pain from a stimulus that does not normally cause pain in the absence of FM
- hyperalgesia, an increased sensitivity to pain from various goads that causes persistent pain. A pinprick in the skin results in amplified pain equal to much more than a pinprick. Increased tenderness occurs in the tender points.

Fibromyalgia patients report the pain as profound, and it considerably affects their lives. The pain is considered widespread if it occurs globally, originating from a tissue injury, and affects tender points over the course of time. The different types of pain are[16]:

- widespread, bilateral pain that occurs both above and below the waist
- nonanatomic distribution (global or regional pain), which is fluctuating and itinerant
- diffuse *arthralgia* affects the joints without redness or swelling
- chest pain that presents as a sensation of a heart attack but is different from *angina*
- low back pain due to the compression of the sciatic nerve
- leg cramps, which occur in 40 percent of patients

- generalized stiffness, similar to morning stiffness but reoccurring throughout the day
- temporomandibular joint disorder (TMD) due to contraction of the muscles in the face and jaw, which causes jaw joint pain and affects 25 percent of FM patients
- frequent or aching cramps or spasms that may be severe because of overworked muscles. These spasms cause intense pain. Muscle knots and cramping can be related to trigger points and cause weakness. Muscles spasms or twitches occur in the presence of other symptoms of FM.

Headaches are another type of pain associated with FM. About half of all FM patients report headaches, a tier of pain that includes migraines, tension-type migraines, post-traumatic cranial pain, and pain in the head due to an overdose of medication. About 75 percent of FM patients who register headaches suffer from chronic headaches; headaches due to overuse of medication occur in 8 percent of patients. General headaches are reported in 53 to 82 percent of patients; tension-type headaches affect 35 percent of FM patients. Headaches occur two or more days a week in 53 percent of FM sufferers. Also, in 47 percent of patients, the headache lasts more than twelve hours. In addition to headaches, patients suffer psychological comorbidities (depression and anxiety, for example). Both FM and primary headaches are associated with widespread pain. Isolated migraine is the most often diagnosed, and in 40 percent of patients with migraines, eleven tender points were identified.[17]

Fatigue or poor stamina crops up often in FM patients, presenting in 90 percent of FM cases. It is sometimes unexpected. The patient can feel worse after physical exercise. Fatigue can be structural (abnormalities of the skeleton), muscular (muscle dysfunction), or metabolic (inability to produce energy). There is sometimes no explanation for the fatigue, and the symptoms are persistent or recurrent. Fatigue leads to a decreased activity level. Nonrestorative sleep can lead to fatigue. Fibromyalgia fatigue is characterized by exhaustion, weakness, heaviness, general malaise, debilitating lightheadedness, and sleepiness. The patient's activity drastically drops, and the patient can become bedridden due to the overwhelming lack of stamina essential to perform daily activities and routines, including work. Severe muscle weakness leads to chronic fatigue. The patient feels tired and exhausted the whole day long. The muscles do not get the necessary supply of energy, and the patient's life is terribly affected. The muscles become tender, and touching them causes a strong ache. Although the muscles are weak, what causes more discomfort is the pain this disease brings to the sufferer's everyday life. Fibromyalgia pain is considered the primary symptom, and the weakness is considered secondary but not any less critical. Fatigue may become severe, leading to poor concentration.[18]

Fibromyalgia causes muscle spasms—involuntary painful contractions of the muscle cells. These spasms initiate low back pain and headaches, but they can occur in any muscle. It has been shown that many FM patients have a change in the mitochondria of the muscle cells, quirks in the blood circulation in these cells, and irregular metabolism, which all lead the way to muscle spasms.[19]

The pain can lead to depression, stress, insomnia, and total loss of energy. It becomes very difficult to manage a normal life in pain, especially when compounded by sleep disorders and chronic fatigue. Social life is furrowed, and FM pain and other symptoms can lead to suicide.[20]

RESPIRATORY SYMPTOMS OF FIBROMYALGIA

Many patients report "fibro breathing" or breathing difficulty.[21]

- Periodic breathing during sleep occurrence is often caused by a reduction of carbon monoxide transfer through the lungs. A significant reduction of the alveolar membrane occurs with a poor sleep condition. Fibromyalgia patients have less slow wave sleep due to pain.
- Exertional dyspnea (shortness of breath with exertion) is very common. The pulmonary causes are unexplained but are probably due to chest wall discomfort and pain.
- Breathing irregularities and breathing dysregulations or attacks of breathlessness may occur on spur of the moment.
- Shortness of breath, when the patient becomes breathless without exertion, is present in 50 percent of patients.
- Shallow breathing (difficulties when taking deep breaths) occur.

- Air hunger, with or without exercise, is common in the majority of FM patients.
- About half of FM patients report chaotic breathing or disordered breathing. The patient can use exercises to relearn correct breathing.
- FM patients often take only small breaths when exercising the abdominal muscles, causing anxiety and pain.

DIGESTIVE SYMPTOMS OF FIBROMYALGIA[22]

- Abdominal cramps can occur in abdominal muscles.
- Bloating and increased gas are usually due to irritable bowel syndrome.
- Decreased appetite is more common in women, more frequent after age fifty, and it is severe in 60 percent of cases.
- Food cravings may arise.
- *Hypoglycemia* occurs in 30 percent of female patients and in 20 percent of male fibromyalgia sufferers. Sugar addiction must be treated.
- Frequent constipation, related to irritable bowel syndrome, is more frequent in women, and it is more common after age fifty. Constipation is severe in 48 percent of cases.
- Chronic heartburn (gastroesophageal reflux or GERD) often occurs with insomnia in many FM patients. The symptoms are belching and an upset stomach. The common medications for FM worsen heartburn, so it must be treated with acid-blocking drugs. A bland diet is often prescribed, and patients are advised to avoid eating too close to bedtime. Weight loss and exercise are also recommended.
- FM patients often report increased appetite and weight gain. Fibromyalgia interferes with leptin, an appetite hormone, and causes it to work irregularly. The patient gains weight because he eats more due to an erroneous signaling message from leptin to the brain.
- Slowed digestion is common in fibromyalgia patients. Weight gain is a common problem, even if they do not overeat. This kind of weight gain is due to lack of sleep, which causes a diminution in metabolism and upturns the appetite for high carb and high-sugar foods. Hor-

mone deficiencies (neuroendocrine abnormalities) increase sensitivity to insulin and decrease metabolism.

- Irritable bladder occurs in 40 to 60 percent of FM patients. This syndrome can cause recurrent urinary tract infections, interstitial cystitis, and gynecological disorders. The symptoms are discomfort with the need to urinate frequently both during the day and at night. Bladder dysfunctions are associated with pain sensitivity and *allodynia*. The cause may be an overgrowth of bacteria in the small intestine due to FM.

- Irritable bowel syndrome (IBS) occurs in 60 percent of FM patients. The syndrome causes abdominal pain, constipation, diarrhea, and alternating disturbance. Evacuation alleviates the symptoms. IBS occurs in the large bowel, but many patients suffer problems in the stomach and small bowel. The symptoms include nausea; abdominal bloating; a constant feeling of fullness; a sensation of heaviness in the stomach; upper- and mid-abdominal pain; belching; and occasional vomiting. Irritable bowel syndrome is a very common gastrointestinal disorder. The syndrome can accompany nongastrointestinal symptoms, such as skin rashes, headaches, and myalgias. Both FM and IBS are functional pain disorders, materializing most often in women, especially with stress, disturbed sleep, and fatigue. Irritable bowel syndrome is intestinal, and FM is somatic. Patients with both diseases suffer increased pain sensation (somatic hyperalgesia). Patients afflicted with IBS have an altered response to somatic and visceral pain because of how the brain processes visceral information with greater responses in pain zones.

- Nausea due to IBS often occurs together with dizziness, sweating, and blurred vision. The patient can feel an urgent need to vomit due to anxiety and stress. The symptoms of nausea are: dizziness, sweating, chills, feeling faint, breathing difficulties, and heart palpitations. It affects between 40 and 70 percent of FM patients. It impairs the routine and lifestyle. Alcohol must be avoided to quell symptoms. The patient struggles to have a normal life, and self-esteem is often compromised.

- Frequent diarrhea and intestinal dysfunction occur in 90 percent of FM patients, and it is often related to anxiety.

- Vomiting is occasional, occurring along with the IBS symptom of feeling full even if the patient has only eaten a small portion of food, and the sensation of fullness leads to vomiting.
- *Interstitial cystitis* also presents in some FM patients, leading to constant urinating. No bacteria is found, although the condition is similar to a bladder infection. Pain in the bladder is constant, and the use of antibiotics actually worsens the bladder pain. It can be present in men and women, but it is seen more frequently in females. The cause is still uncharted. Interstitial cystitis is rare, and the diagnosis is therefore difficult to determine. Cranberry juice worsens the condition because it accelerates pain and spasms. It is recommended that patients drink plenty of water and follow an adequate diet. It can be treated with a catheter, and a prescription for Elavil, an antidepressant, can alleviate the pain. Consumption of citrus fruits, chocolate, and alcohol must be greatly reduced or eliminated to reduce the chances of recurrence.
- Intestinal irregularities and bladder dysfunction are frequent in FM patients. Moreover, substance P and serotonin play an important role in the development of the symptoms. Patients feel the need to urinate as frequently as every twenty minutes. Such repeated trips to the bathroom can flail life quality and self-esteem. It impairs relations in daily life. It is due to an overactive or irritable bladder, affected by nerves and muscles.
- Painful urination presents with a chronic ache and difficulty urinating. It can also occur with bladder pain and prostate pain. Also, FM patients and caregivers should note that bladder dysfunction is associated with allodynia and pain.

Changes in weather, lack of exercise, rest instability, stress, anxiety, and depression can aggravate the symptoms of FM. They vary from mild to severe. All of these symptoms must be treated with the correct medication and lifestyle modification. The symptoms can become severe but are not life threatening. All of the symptoms can be alleviated, but some will never be completely relieved.[23]

All in all, FM has many symptoms. Patients may experience some or all of the symptoms. They can vary from patient to patient. Many of the systematic symptoms are connected, and the severity of the symptoms can fluctuate over time. Fibromyalgia symptoms are likely to be chronic. Sleep disturbance is a primary characteristic of FM. Headaches, especially migraines, occur commonly in FM patients. The main and most persistent symptom of FM is musculoskeletal pain, but it can cause other significant symptoms, including those of the nervous system, respiratory tract, and gastrointestinal regions. Sleep is indefectible against FM, and nonrestorative sleep can lead to intense fatigue, which aggravates this painful condition. Resilient snooze is great for the treatment of FM since the latter is known to be a chronic and painful condition affecting many sites of the body.[24]

II

Clinical Picture

4

BRAIN FOG: MYTH OR REALITY?

Brain fog is a term that describes brain complications as experienced by patients with fibromyalgia (FM) with respect to cognitive capacity, mental malaise, mental confusion and forgetfulness, and reoccurring problems of concentration and attention caused by a dearth of sleep. It impedes the FM patient from processing information. The individual becomes forgetful, cloudy, and has difficulty concentrating, focusing, communicating, and thinking. In essence, the brain functions slacken. Brain fog is similar to mental fatigue. The causes may be physical, emotional, or biochemical, but researchers have not yet confirmed the true derivation of fibro fog. It is possible that brain fog or fibro fog is caused by FM pain. It is known that fibro fog is connected with an imbalance in the nervous system. Cortisol can cause brain damage, impairing memory. Allergies (especially food allergies) and hormonal disturbances can cause brain fog, and they must be treated to reduce the fog. Excessive consumption of caffeine and alcohol may cause brain fog. There are medications—for example, sleeping pills—that prompt memory loss.[1]

Brain fog, or fibro fog, occurs mainly in women (approximately 90 percent of female patients) and after the age of forty. Fibro fog is more frequently seen in patients after age fifty. The symptoms are moderate but negatively affect quality of life and can include[2]:

- mental malaise
- mental confusion and forgetfulness

- problems with concentration and attention caused by a lack of sleep
- impaired focus, attention, and concentration
- problems with memory and concentration capacity
- dyslexia (difficulty reading letters and symbols)

The patient should make lifestyle changes to muddle through brain fog. Good-quality sleep is important to oppose the fibro fog. Caffeine and alcohol must be avoided. It is also important that the patient focus on just one task at a time to preclude confusion. To avoid the fibro fog, and for its treatment, brain exercises are often necessary. What's more, reading interesting subjects helps battle the symptoms. Good blood supply, adequate blood quantity, strong *neurotransmitters*, and sufficient oxygen are also necessary to avoid fogginess.[3]

Brain fog is very common in women during menopause due to hormone ups and downs, similar to the "pregnancy brain" felt by pregnant women and new mothers. Other triggers of brain fog that can be controlled or eliminated include[4]:

- nutrient deficiencies, especially calcium, magnesium, B complex, zinc, selenium, omega-3 fatty acids, and proteins
- lack of sleep or rest
- bowel toxicity
- Yin disease, due to consuming fruit and sugar
- dehydration
- reactions to foods or its additives and supplements, such as aspartame and aspartic acid
- prolonged standing
- a fainting sensation

Toxic metals, such as copper, mercury, lead, aluminum, nickel, and cadmium, are other grating triggers. Excessive copper causes confusion and disorientation and affects the thyroid glands, which all are catalysts of brain fog. Copper imbalance leads to an overabundance of candida and can lead to yeast infections. Sauna therapy is good for removing toxic metals. Drugs and medications can also be noxious to a certain extent, such as medication for allergies, pain, blood pressure, heart arrhythmia, depression, anxiety, and inflammation. In cancer patients, chemotherapy creates an immense risk for the development of fibro fog. Environmental toxins play a large role in the occurrence of the disorder: heavy metals, *phthalates*, insecticides, and pesticides are mitochondrial toxins. Last, mitochondria produces adenosine triphosphate, which is responsible for the cognitive health of brain cells.[5]

Stress is a focal trigger of brain fog. Stress must be managed and future stressful situations must be avoided to raze the chances of recurring fog. Exercises such as walking have proven beneficial in the struggle against the disorder. Brain stress is a trigger factor of brain fog. Brain tumors, epilepsy, meningitis, and encephalitis can also cause brain fog.[6]

Moreover, reduced oxygen in the brain can be due to clogged arteries, low blood pressure, and shallow breathing. Asthma, chronic bronchitis, and emphysema ruin breathing processes. Electromagnetic stress is set off by the use of mobile devices, overuse of computers, or watching TV at a near distance. Poor blood circulation is due to low blood pressure and arteriosclerosis, while drugs such as marijuana and alcohol cause brain damage. All of these triggers must be eliminated in order to relegate the fog.[7]

Fibro fog worsens the otherwise smooth execution of tasks, such as those at work, school, and home. Productivity usually decreases. Anxiety and depression also often occur in patients with fibro fog. Fibromyalgia fog patients have a higher incidence of brain fog than nonpatients, and it can be considered an early/mild dementia state, although it is actually poles apart from true dementia. Studies have shown that memory deteriorates with FM. Brain fog involves mental fogginess and memory loss, and the patient loses track of the evolvement of a task, such as reading, TV watching, and speaking. The person has difficulty expressing himself or simply communicating. Absentmindedness is typical in brain fog along with forgetfulness, concentration problems, disorientation, and other cognitive difficulties. Vestibular abnormalities (difficulty controlling balance and eye movements) are associated with fibro fog. Moreover, sensitivity to light and noise and spatial disorientation are also associated with brain fog. Inflammation, such as inflammation in the gums around the teeth, can be a hidden trigger. Fibromyalgia patients and caregivers should also note that spinal misalignment must be remedied and corrected to prevent additional brain fog. Traumas and mental problems must also be addressed. Brain fog causes chronic constipation, diarrhea, and inflammatory disease.[8]

Memory loss is perhaps the most frustrating side effect as it impairs daily routine. Things such as forgetting where keys or documents are are very annoying. Difficulty remembering a person's name can be very embarrassing. The patient often has the sensation that he is losing his mind. These cognitive dysfunctions are very stressful, leading to difficulties in family and social life. At work, forgetting how to do routine tasks makes things complicated. Difficulty speaking, finding the correct words, and following along with a conversation may lead to a very frustrating emplacement among friends. Cognitive abilities are essential to have a normal life at home, at work, and at school. The patient feels that the brain is "aging" faster than the body and does not work as well as it should for its actual age.[9]

It is very stressful to forget an appointment with the doctor or with children's teachers, or the correct word choice in response to a question; these all create stressful situations. Forgetting important data can lead to costly results, both in terms of life, health, and finances. For example, consider a patient who works at a school and receives a call that the water supply will be interrupted the following day. This is important information that must be relayed to the principal. If the FM patient does not remember to pass on the information, the principal cannot take the necessary measures. The students and staff will be without water, and this will create a difficult situation for everyone involved. Memory, information, and communication are focal aspects of a normal life, and their impairment causes frustration and stress. The patient must adopt the habit of noting the main tasks that must be done during the day. Making notes helps coordinate the flow of the tasks and helps keep the patient from losing track. Essentially, the person who does not communicate gets in trouble. This trouble may have serious consequences for the patient, family members, work colleagues, and classmates alike.[10]

For all of these symptoms and the problems that fibro fog causes, the trouble-free treatment or solution is adequate exercise, medication, and diet. There are several behavior modifications that can help reduce fibro fog, including developing a routine for significant tasks, avoiding distractions, double-checking numbers and words, and avoiding medications that cause dizziness. If the fibro fog is astringent, the patient must not drive. Being organized helps the patient stay on track, which is important when trying to overcome brain fog. Relaxation is a good remedy against fibro fog, as are exercises such as walking and aquatic exercise, and they must be included in treatment. Yoga, tai chi, and meditation are good treatments. Memory techniques are helpful against brain fog, and crossword puzzles and logic puzzles can activate the brain. Meditation helps in dealing with stress, which can reactivate cognition. Avoiding sensitivity triggers is important to improve the patient's overall health. Brain fog can be treated, and the patient must look for professional, psychological, and medical assistance. Detoxification procedures, such as using a sauna or two daily coffee enemas, are also advocated.[11]

The treatment for brain fog includes herbs, homeopathic supplements, vitamins, minerals, hormones, and prescription medications. The patient must be careful using any of these treatments because they can sometimes worsen the symptoms instead of amending them. A diet rich in nutrients is essential to moderating the symptoms of fibro fog. The patient must avoid the foods that are known to trigger fibro fog, including sugar and products containing sugar such as soda and sweets, white bread, pasta, and white rice. The patient's diet should contain food without chemicals. Brain supplements are likewise favorable in the treatment of brain fog, such as omega-3 fatty acid supplements, vitamin B12 and vitamin D, high-quality antioxidant formula multivitamins, and multi-ingredient brain supplements. Ribose, a natural sugar, should be included in the regimen because it improves clarity. A diet with oil is advisable (lecithin, coconut oil, or hemp oil); organic oil is important for the immune system.[12]

HOW THE TERM *BRAIN FOG* (OR *FIBRO FOG*) CAME TO BE USED

The term *brain fog* largely came to be used with the study of the development of FM in the 1990s. This term is not the most accurate, but it is the word most often wrought within circles of conversation. The appurtenant term is *cognitive dysfunction*. Fibro fog is not a medically recognized disorder but rather a condition. The symptoms are very real and present, but fibro fog is not considered a true disease. Brain fog is not considered an official symptom of FM because cognitive dysfunction can sometimes be related to an inflammation in the brain.

As it is largely studied, inflammation does not occur in all fibro patients, so brain fog (as related to a brain inflammation) cannot be considered a symptom of FM. As already explained, the main characteristic for FM is pain and not inflammation.[13]

BENEFITS AND DRAWBACKS OF USING BROAD, VAGUE THEORIES IN MEDICINE

Health is not exclusively biological, and neither is brain fog. Health is a combination of biological, psychological, and social factors. There is immense criticism of using broad, vague theories in medicine. Theories are ideas, and while they are often standardized, they are speculations, after all. Nonetheless, the benefit of a theory is that it brings about an explanation, for example, of the possible causes of a disease. It opens the door to further research. The science, in general, begins with a philosophical theory; if the medical science, through examination, verification, and research, certifies the reality of such a theory, then it will become a confirmed fact. The proof is a fact, such as a disease, first based on a theory. The drawback of a profoundly cursory theory is that it has no scientific confirmation. It is just speculation, a probability, or a possibility of what an issue might be. Until confirmation, the theories undergo severe criticism and are perceived by many scientists as controversial. Without actual proof, medical science cannot assert the theory (i.e., brain fog before it was positively identified) as confirmed truth. Many theories come to confirmation and become respected as fact and accepted as real and fundamental by the medical society in its totality.[14]

Science is dynamic. Researchers and scientists are curious and eager for information, and explanations and the need to know leads to questioning the possibilities and probabilities of issues in all areas of knowledge. Without theories, medical science stagnates, and does not develop and change and does not reach enough progress to find out whether possibilities have veracity. Vague theories can, in a scientific domain, speak about many other theories that have not found scientific confirmation of its truth as a scientific fact. If the researchers and scientists do not exercise speculation, looking for conceivable solutions and truths, science, as well as medical science, remains vegetated, and new discoveries cannot be made. The vague and broad theories, such as those pertaining to brain fog, are the first steps to getting the information that is needed for, in this case, the scientific confirmation of a severe disease. Many theories remain without confirmation, but if scientists make every effort to prove or disprove a theory, the possibility can turn into a real fact, a real disease, and progress will be made so that development is achieved. Progress in the field of fibromyalgia opens new doors to medical knowledge. Many theories are corroborated with proof. Other theories are overcome with new findings, and their probability is eliminated. This is the way of progress in science. Many possibilities become facts proven through scientific research. Without asking why, answers that satisfy the need of knowing the causes and effects of a matter such as fibro fog cannot be unearthed. In medicine, it occurs the same way—physicians and researchers are enthusiastic to know more and more about the diseases occurring in the world, but many things remain wrapped in mystery and supposition.[15]

Fibro fog is definitely associated with FM, but it is not an official symptom acknowledged for diagnosis. That is perhaps why *fibro fog*, a term largely used since the 1990s with the development of the study of FM, is more appropriately called *cognitive dysfunction*. Fibro fog is not recognized as a disease, but it is real, and the symptoms can be severe. It affects the brain, causing memory loss and concentration-related quagmires. The symptoms can be alleviated through proper relaxation and shuteye. It greatly affects the patient's life in the family and in society, as it equally causes problems at school and at work. It is important to look for professional, psychological, and medical assistance.[16]

5

CAUSES OF FIBROMYALGIA

Fibromyalgia sufferers often have a hyperactive lifestyle before a diagnosis is made. The patient's anxiety can lead to hyperactivity. The FM patient cannot find the relief from the symptoms of the disease and can become anxious and panicky. The absence of adequate rest makes the situation even worse. Hyperactivity often leads to maladies such as FM.

It is important to maintain a healthy lifestyle, limiting alcohol, caffeine, and poor food choices. All these activities and others with a negative impact ought to be jettisoned so that the patient can achieve a high quality of life and get control of the symptoms of this disease. The patient can gain control by following basic self-care guidelines to successfully live with FM[1]:

- Reduce stress. It is important to have balance and avoid overexertion and emotional stress. The patient must avoid feeling guilty and, if possible, should continue to work because life without activity aggravates the symptoms of FM.
- Patients should strive to regulate sleep hours and avoid daytime napping. Sleep disturbance and fatigue is common in FM because of a lack of sleep or bad quality of sleep.
- Exercise, always exercise, slowly, but without overexerting. Exercise may upheave the pain in the beginning, but if the exercise routine is built up gradually, the pain will subside and the symptoms will lessen. Recommended exercises include walking, swimming, biking, and water exercises. A physical therapist or doctor

can choose the best options and will also include therapies such as stretching and relaxation.

- Pacing is expedient, and moderation is the key for the success of the treatment.

Incorporating lifestyle changes is the single most important measure that must be taken in the treatment of FM, and a long-term exercise program is essential for effective treatment. The patient must strive to manage a satisfying life and overall well-being, which will gradually improve the patient's condition and help overcome pain and fatigue, the main symptoms of the disease. A good sleep routine will lead the patient to a good quality of life. This can be obtained through an exercise program that includes aerobics, strength training, and flexibility exercises. Exercise coupled with education on FM, its symptoms and causes, plus a balanced diet will help tremendously. The most sanctioned exercise for this disorder is called graded exercise, which involves a soft beginning that gradually increases until reaching the level necessary to combat the symptoms. It has been shown that stretching is powerful in the treatment of FM as it leads to muscle relaxation and alleviates pain. Exercises such as swimming and water therapy are beneficial in the control of the disease because they do not impair the joints. Difficult or strenuous exercises must be evaded because they can worsen the symptoms of the illness and are not beneficial in the treatment result. In everyday life, the patient must cope with symptoms that are recurrent. A physical therapist can assess the best exercise that fits the needs of the individual patient, as the disease varies from patient to patient. Physical therapy has proven effective in the treatment of FM.[2]

WHO IS AT AN INCREASED RISK FOR FIBROMYALGIA?

In order to fathom the various steps or actions that can be taken for the prevention of FM, it is important for patients and caregivers to understand who exactly is at risk. This is a disorder that affects more women than men, but apart from gender there are several other factors that can determine the onset of FM[3]:

- Age is a palmary indicator that a doctor should consider an FM diagnosis. This disorder normally occurs more often in women, but it can occur in men as well. There are a few rare cases of FM occurring in elderly people as well as in children. The average age at onset disclosed by a research study is thirty-five. The fact is that if an individual older than thirty-five has the symptoms of FM, then there is a high probability of FM and a diagnosis must be determined by following up with tests and medication.
- Family medical history is another factor that contributes to FM. If this disorder occurs anywhere else in the family tree, even if the person afflicted is a distant relative, the diagnosis cannot be ruled out. There will always be the risk of picking up the disorder.
- Other rheumatic diseases can instigate FM. Those who are already suffering from some form of rheumatic disorder or disease such as lupus or rheumatoid arthritis are at a higher risk for developing FM than others in the same age group.
- Stress, as suggested by certain studies, can contribute to the onset of FM. Studies also hint that people with stressful or traumatic life experiences are also at a higher risk of getting FM.[4]

FATIGUE AND ITS ROLE IN FIBROMYALGIA

Fatigue can crop up on anyone and can be caused by several factors. Fatigue is an extreme form of tiredness that gets in the way of completing basic tasks or daily activities. Chronic fatigue can put a person at a higher risk for several medical conditions including FM. This type of prolonged tiredness can be psychological, emotional, or physical in nature and can limit a person's ability to execute tasks at work or home. It can be from lack of sleep, a hectic workload, too much stress, or even traumatic events.

PHYSICAL AND MENTAL STRESS AND FIBROMYALGIA

The FM patient must cope with emotions. Fibromyalgia causes so much pain that it often leads the patient to gain psychiatric disorders such as depression and anxiety, and it is something the patient must face in daily life. Fibromyalgia patients often undergo chronic depression. In this case, the patient must pursue the professional help of a psychologist to help balance emotions and for copacetic mental health. The role of family and friends is essential to helping the patient overcome the devastating emotional impact of FM. Patients are advised to join support groups that will help connect them with other FM patients. The treatment of the depression caused by FM is long and must be approached with dedication and effort. One alternative therapy for depression is *cognitive behavioral therapy*, which is also excellent in handling of anxiety. It is effective and reduces pain.[5]

Anxiety can present as a generalized anxiety disorder, which causes the following[6]:

- fear, panic, muscle aches, and fatigue
- depression wherein the patient walks anxiously in circles instead of lying in bed
- a chronic-panic disorder, which is characterized by panic attacks, profuse sweating, and the sensation of a heart attack
- obsessive-compulsive disorder, which causes the patients to perform repetitive tasks such as hand washing and counting
- post-traumatic stress disorder, which makes the patient relive past traumatic experiences such as rape, childhood abuse, or combat venues

Anxiety can be treated with relaxation therapy and medication.

The absence of relaxation such as going on vacation, catching a movie, and performing enjoyable activities can lead to stress. Sometimes the person looks for relaxation from the improper source, such as with the use of alcohol. It is undeniable that physical and mental stress deteriorates the FM patient's condition. The pain becomes chronic; stress does not cause pain but it worsens the already existing pain. In the course of a day, many activities can lead the patient to stress either at work or at home. When stressed, the patient can become nervous and tend to criticize family members or friends. If the patient wakes up feeling stressed, it would be prudent to start the day with meditation or other relaxing activities. If daily activities spike the stress level, the patient should take a break, try to relax, and once calm resume the task at hand. The stress sufferer often has the sensation that other people are too demanding or are working in opposition to them.[7]

Consider this scenario of a FM patient at work. The boss assigns an additional task to a person with FM. Fibromyalgia patients can often feel laden and consider their supervisor and colleagues unsympathetic. The FM patient might react in anger or "explode." In a stressful situation like this, the patient feels alone, abandoned, and believes family, friends, and colleagues don't care. The patient often begins to feel helpless and lonely. The stressed FM patient might regard immediate family and friends as encumbrances. The person tends to develop a negative outlook and may abuse alcohol. The patient's sleep disturbance worsens the situation, and anxiety and depression begin to dominate.[8]

Relaxation therapy is recommended to head off these kinds of scenarios. The patient must calm both body and mind in order to find stress relief. Regular use of relaxation therapy and its techniques can lead to stress reduction or elimination. When a person is under stress, blood pressure rises and aggravates the other symptoms of FM. It is recommended to go seek the help of a therapist and become involved in talk therapy.[9]

The patient must take time to rest, relax, and forget the daily routine with its storms. Listening to soothing music is a good practice. The person must learn to take time to appreciate nature—the birds, the animals, the landscapes, and other parts of the environment—to find relaxation and to eliminate both physical and mental stress. Activities such as meditation, yoga, and tai chi have demonstrated efficacy in the treatment of physical and mental stress. Without stress, the FM patient's condition improves both physically and intellectually. Family members can play a significant role by avoiding adding stress to the patient. The patient must tweak his sleep condition to reduce stress levels. Sleep disturbances such as insomnia must be treated not with medications alone but also with lifestyle changes, including affixing exercises to the daily routine.[10]

Hypnosis, an alternative treatment for stress, works for some patients with FM. It leads to a better sleep, reduces fatigue, and alleviates other FM symptoms. The patient must look for the best hypnotherapist to eliminate stress. There are techniques the patient can learn to use to accomplish self-hypnosis without the need of a professional.[11]

Stress reduction activities include meditation and yoga. Meditation relieves pain, reduces depression, and improves sleep. Yoga is beneficial for improving the patient's condition, but it should be done unhurriedly to avoid pain and strain. The patient with FM must cope with stress and minimize it as stress triggers FM symptoms. Managing stress can eliminate or reduce depression, anxiety, fatigue, and above all lead to good sleep quality. The stress sprung from emotions must be treated and arrangements must be made at work to curtail stress situations. Many FM patients demonstrate a stress history in the development of the disease, so FM can be considered as the result of a stressful experience.[12]

Some researchers do not consider stress as a primary factor in the occurrence of the disease, although it plays a significant role in its development. In patients with FM, stress worsens the condition both physically and mentally, leading to more pain and anxiety. The more relaxed the person is, the less FM symptoms the patient reports.[13]

CULTURAL, ENVIRONMENTAL, AND GENETIC FACTORS OF FIBROMYALGIA

Cultural and environmental factors are not too prominent in FM, but they do contribute to the disease. These factors make the person susceptible to the disease; they are involved in the trigger of FM and, worse, they perpetuate the disease. Social and family factors, both emotional and physical, impact the life of patients, such as sexual abuse by family members or spouses. Studies have demonstrated that rape victims develop FM with more frequency. Relatives of FM patients are more susceptible to developing the disease than other persons not related to a patient. Family members are more sensitive to pain, and can acquire disorders related to FM such as irritable bowel syndrome, headaches, and jaw pain (temporomandibular disorder). Risk factors include originating from a stressful culture or environment, being prone to stress, and having had bad experiences as a child. A person susceptible to the disease living in a stressful environment is more likely to develop FM.[14]

The absolute role of genetic factors in FM is still wrapped in uncertainty and remains a mystery, but it is clear that genes somehow play an expressive role in the development of the disease. The genetically prone family member is likely to develop FM if exposed to a stressful environment or culture. Genetic data as a risk factor are more inferential than definitive, so if the person is genetically predisposed to have FM it does not necessarily denote that FM will develop and the person will suffer the disease. Environmental and cultural factors may contribute to the development of the disease in genetically prone individuals. Without stressful cultural or environment factors, the genetic risk of contracting FM is minimal.[15]

In summary, the risk factors of contracting FM can be cultural, environmental, and genetic. Family members are more vulnerable to FM than the general population. A stressful culture and surroundings is not a primary cause, but it is no less instrumental in the incidence of the disease.[16]

6

OUTPATIENT VS. INPATIENT CARE IN FIBROMYALGIA TREATMENT

Fibromyalgia (FM) patients with mild to chronic cases need not be hospitalized to receive proper care and treatment. These FM patients are treated by their physicians on an outpatient basis, and they can lodge in their home environment and perform almost all usual undertakings. The patient can enroll in a restorative care program that provides support and services for recovery. These settings typically last about eight weeks and focus on the treatment of the symptoms.

FIBROMYALGIA OUTPATIENT CARE

Along with medical care, the program educates the patient on the disorder, symptoms, treatments, and self-care. These programs encourage the patient to perform self-management techniques that help oust the symptoms of the illness and the psychiatric and psychological effects the disorder causes. Education is often based on physical therapy, integrating education, exercise, aquatic therapy, tai chi, and neural integration. The American College of Rheumatology recommend these exercises to focus on alleviating pain and fatigue and improving sleep and mood quality. Aquatic therapy is urged for patients who fear exercises that require strain and exacerbate their pain. Tai chi and neural integration therapy abate symptoms of FM and increase flexibility, balance, and strength and provide improvement in the quality of life. The program team recommending these treatments is comprised of physicians and physical therapists.[1]

The medical department at the University of Pittsburgh developed an animal-assisted therapy study using dogs that were trained to help the patient, and the results were positive for individuals with FM. The patients felt better with the dogs' presence in the waiting room, resulting in a prevailing improvement in health. It is a complementary treatment for outpatients and results in a meaningful reduction of pain and distress. In general, the outpatient receives medical treatment, psychological support, and education.[2]

A patient who does not need a hospital stay is still able to get the necessary care and is oriented to perform exercise therapy. The physician provides proper medication. The patient is taught to perform self-care. This kind of treatment is salutary, and the result is positive. The goal is to prevent the patient from aggravating an already dilapidated mental and physical health. Every effort is made so that the sufferer has no need to remain in the hospital with constant care.[3]

FIBROMYALGIA INPATIENT CARE

Fibromyalgia patients with severe cases need medical care on an inpatient basis at the hospital. Patients with mild to chronic cases can be treated on an outpatient basis and receive the needed medical care at the doctor's office and can perform some self-care treatments at home. Today it is not difficult to find the right doctor to treat FM because there is an immeasurable variety of professionals and therapies that can bring pain relief and improve the health condition of FM patients. The patient must find the most adequate doctor or therapist. The diagnosis is made primarily by a rheumatologist, but other physicians can treat the disease and its large variety of symptoms and complications. The patient must feel comfortable with the specialist, so he must choose the most appropriate one. Time is required to find the right one.[4]

The patient who needs to be hospitalized must receive constant medical care. Hospitalization is carried out in severe cases of the disease, when the patient is in no condition to perform self-care. The patient receives the necessary medical treatment for FM and is taught how to accomplish self-care once well enough to be discharged from the hospital. Studies show that chest pain is the leading reason for emergency room visits by FM patients.[5]

FINDING THE RIGHT DOCTOR FOR FIBROMYALGIA MANAGEMENT

Finding a fitting doctor to treat FM can be very time consuming. The specialist must believe that FM is in fact a real disease. Until recent years, FM was not considered a true disease, and some doctors believed the condition only existed in the patient's mind. Some physicians still doubt the validity of the illness. The FM diagnosis is often made by a rheumatologist, a primary care doctor, or a neurologist. The primary care doctor can recommend the most appropriate specialist for the patient. Rheumatologists typically treat FM, but there is some debate concerning whether a rheumatologist is the best medical professional to manage FM. Some experts believe FM cases should be treated by a more specialized professional such as a clinical psychologist, pain-management specialist, or primary care physician because it is not a rheumatic disease. Fibromyalgia can also be treated by primary care doctors, podiatrists, osteopaths, homeopaths, neurologists, psychiatrists, and nurse practitioners. Physical therapists can treat some symptoms of FM. Occupational therapists, on the other hand, can expung stress attached to the medical condition. Speech therapists treat patients with fibro fog. For the treatment of FM, the professional must be qualified and intermingle with a team that can provide the necessary care for those hurting from FM.[6]

There are many medical specialists who can treat FM. Among them, a family practice physician offers general medical care for all ages, including preventative health care and care for acute and chronic diseases. Many family practice physicians are ideal for the treatment of FM. A neurologist treats diseases of the nervous system, such as the brain, spinal cord, nerves, and muscles and also treats headaches, migraines, and restless leg syndrome. A gastroenterologist treats the digestive organs such as the stomach, liver, intestines, and gallbladder, and is specialized in the diseases of the abdomen, including pain, ulcers, diarrhea, constipation, irritable bowel syndrome, and gut illnesses. An osteopath performs surgery and prescribes medications with attention to joints, bones, muscles, and nerves. An allergist-immunologist deals with diseases of the immune system, including asthma, *rhinitis*, and eczema. A pain management specialist can be an anesthesiologist, neurologist, psychiatrist, or psychologist, and provides more than primary care. A pain management specialist works together with other specialists. A psychiatrist's goal is to restore functions, whereas an orthopedist specializes in diagnosing and treating diseases such as FM. He also performs surgical repairs for bone injuries. He treats *tendons*, *ligaments*, *cartilage*, and muscle and joint disorders.

When choosing a formal caregiver such as a physician, the patient must consider:

- Is the professional specialized in FM?
- Does the doctor treat patients with FM?
- Does the provider work with a team?
- Does the patient feel comfortable with the doctor?
- Does the doctor pay attention when the patient is relating symptoms?
- Is the doctor's office conveniently located near the patient's home or workplace?

Not all FM doctors will properly dissever the patient's needs from wants. The patient must keep looking for the right doctor, asking the same questions each time until finding positive answers. The patient must consider that this relationship with the doctor will be for a long time, even possibly lifelong, so the most appropriate specialist must be discerned. The patient must have a positive view toward the care provider. The professional must have experience in treating FM, be willing to cooperate with the patient and other providers such as therapists, and must be empathetic and comprehensive. A good starting point to finding the right doctor is to speak to other patients who have FM and have had good results with their doctor. The patient must consider that the right doctor toils for the harmony of medicine.[7]

A professional who loves the chosen career field will do it accordingly and with accuracy. A hue of commitment to "practice and patient" is realistically the doctor's behavior toward his client: a stalwart professional works with dedication, listens to the patient's complaints with attention, and strives to promote the best solution for the patient's condition. An FM doctor who works just for money does not perform the duties of the profession in the same manner, does not pay attention to patients, and constantly seeks more patients than necessary to keep the business teeming. Medicine is a very lucrative field, and some professionals work with the goal of becoming wealthy. The professional who thinks only in terms of money views the patients as only a number, a lane to meet the goal of becoming wealthy.[8]

The patient must be confident and comfortable with the chosen doctor. The doctor will be providing the necessary health and lifestyle care the patient needs. The patient must also trust in the new doctor because some symptoms will require the patient to discuss intimate particulars. So in choosing the right doctor, the patient must trust the doctor completely. There are physicians who do not provide a sense of aplomb to the patient. One tip to discover whether the patient can trust a doctor is hearing the doctor speak about other patients. If the professional speaks of other patients and reveals their secrets, the doctor cannot be trusted. Finding an apposite doctor may require time, but it really does pay to search.[9]

Patients can also find guidance from medical professionals outside of the physician loop. A pharmacist can help the patient with information about prescriptions, including drug interactions and side effects. Nurses who work with the physicians can administer medications and monitor side effects. They can be very helpful in the treatment of diseases, including FM.[10]

A physical therapist helps the patient in the restoration of functions, in the improvement of mobility, and, most importantly for FM patients, they placate pain. A physical therapist teaches the patient exercises such as stretching, muscle strengthening, and motion exercises. The goal of the physical therapist is to foster body fitness using a large variety of methods such as tests, strength measure, balance, and coordination. A registered dietician helps the patient find an adequate nutrition plan in accordance with the patient's current health condition and symptoms.[11]

Furthermore, an acupuncturist uses needles to alleviate pain, but a massage therapist uses massage with varying degrees of pressure to help diminish pain and induce relaxation. An aquatic therapist works with the patient through a large variety of water techniques. Techniques include ai chi (water therapy combining yoga and tai chi) and watsu (passive water therapy).[12]

An occupational therapist works on the social, emotional, and psychological effects of a disease, providing the patient with the ability to have a normal life. Behavioral health professionals include psychologists, as well as psychiatrists, who are in fact physicians. In FM cases, behavioral health experts deal with depression and mental health. A psychologist treats feelings and emotions, such as depression, stress, and anxiety. A psychologist is very important in the treatment of FM because the use of cognitive behavioral therapy can help the patient face pain. A psychiatrist treats mental disorders, such as schizophrenia, anxiety, mood disorder, and bipolar disorder. Psychiatrists work in the biological, psychological, and social expanses of disease. For the FM patient, a psychiatrist prescribes the correct medication for the emotional symptoms and provides assistance for the family members facing problems such as stress as an upshot of the loved one's FM.[13]

The patient expects that the doctor chosen to treat FM will provide the correct medication for treatment, evaluate progress in the healing process, provide assistance in urgent cases, and can help with both emotional and physical symptoms. If the doctor does not meet the patient's needs, the patient has the onus to look for another specialist who can provide the necessary succor and care. The important thing is the patient must feel confident with any and all physicians treating the condition. The physician must provide necessary and adequate treatment. If it is difficult for the client to find the right doctor, health associations and organizations can make recommendations and lead the patient to the corresponding specialist.[14]

7

ROLES OF FAMILY PHYSICIANS, INTERNISTS, AND NEUROLOGISTS

It is essential for family physicians to spend more time listening and understanding the everyday struggle that patients face living with such a chronic disease. Physicians should attempt to slash the incidence of the undesirable effects of various symptoms and play a pivotal role in boosting the overall quality of life of the infirmed.[1]

ROLE OF A FAMILY PHYSICIAN

The family physician is often a general practitioner with a minimum of three years of experience in practicing medicine. He boasts an area of specialization in the study of diseases in adults and internal medicine. It is extremely important that after identifying the first symptoms of FM the physician quickly carries out an assessment of the severities of symptoms. In cases in which special treatment or care is required, the doctor needs to ensure the patient is referred to a FM specialist, such as a neurologist or rheumatologist. A family physician is able to recommend a treatment plan, which may or may not entail medication. There are many nondrug treatments that are recommended by family physicians[2]:

- Cognitive behavioral therapy is extremely effective.

- Alternate therapy, often validated by the family physician and conducted at the clinic or premises of a physiotherapist or psychologist, include rehabilitation, relaxation, psychological support, and physiotherapy.
- *Balneotheraphy* (heated pool treatment) helps decrease pain and improve muscle and nerve functioning, and it works best in conjunction with various exercise routines.
- Aerobic exercise and strength training are recommended according to the nature of symptoms and the overall health and fitness of the individual patient and are tailored by family physicians who are aware of the medical history and individual requirements.

New research has purveyed more and more information pertaining to the symptoms of FM. Research has also shown that patients suffering from this disorder often have a deficiency of certain minerals and vitamins. Studies have shown that FM is in many ways linked to a high level of homocysteine, which is an amino acid produced by the body. The new information and findings help physicians better identify and doff the symptoms of FM. If a physician's diagnosis reveals a lack of vitamins or minerals, then a multivitamin can be prescribed. Vitamin and mineral levels must be honed as they are essential for energy release, normal operation of muscles, production of serotonin, and improved functioning of the nervous system.[3]

One of the minerals that is often deficient in those suffering from FM is magnesium. A few tests can be conducted by the family physician to clarify current levels. If any deficiency is observed, then the physician will likely recommend a healthy diet containing seafood, dark green leafy vegetables, nuts, and whole grains.[4]

ROLE OF AN INTERNIST

Internists (internal medicine specialists) deal with adult medicine and have the knowledge to prescribe sundry medications for stabilizing and improving the overall quality of life while also ensuring there are no drug interactions, side effects, or toxicities. The internist is normally the first specialist seen who has the knack to evaluate the symptoms of FM and can effectively provide the required treatment to annul the patient's condition or malaise. The primary goal of an internist is to work with a patient suffering from FM by taking them through three different paths or stages[5]:

- Adequate sleep is one of the most effective treatments for FM, and an internist will work with patients to help them understand and modify their lifestyle and habits to conserve an improved sleep environment and to decrease pain.
- Relief from pain can be achieved through medication, pain modulators, or antidepressants. Medicine can also effectively treat anxiety, depression, and fatigue that often spanned with FM.
- Other therapies can include an exercise plan made up of aerobic exercises, stress reduction, relaxation therapies, moist heat therapy, and other forms of physical therapy.

If the symptoms linger, the internist can refer the patient to any of several specialists[6]:

- Neurologists are specialists who can diagnose as well as treat any disorder involving the nervous system. They have the ability to treat pain-related disorders including FM, headaches, muscle disorders, back pain, and reflex sympathetic dystrophy (RSD).
- Rheumatologists specialize in diagnosis and treatment of diseases and pain associated with bones, muscles, and joints. This includes FM, osteoarthritis, rheumatoid arthritis, and back pain, among others.
- Pain specialists are adept in pain management and can include medical-board-certified neurologists, anesthesiologists, and psychiatrists.
- Orthopedists are bone and joint mavens who can diagnose and offer clinical treatment.
- Psychologists' roles revolve around diagnosing the nature and cause of the disorder and providing effective therapy to mitigate pain, anxiety, and depression.

ROLE OF A NEUROLOGIST IN FM

The indispensable role of a neurologist is to diagnose nervous system disorders and provide the necessary management and treatment. A neurologist is a preferred choice to treat FM, as several symptoms are associated with specific complaints involving the central nervous system (CNS). Researchers believe that FM begins in the brain and is molded by what is known as a pain processing disorder. Since one of the areas of specialization of a neurologist is the CNS, they are arguably the most revered and learned of all medical practitioners to treat FM. Patients are normally advised to visit a neurologist when the symptoms of FM are first diagnosed. Moreover, one of the important functions that a neurologist carries out is to narrow down the primary grounds of pain related to the disorder and then provide treatment. There are several neurologists whose primary focus is to provide relief from different types of pain, including those arising from FM. There are several different ways in which a neurologist can help patients suffering from this medical condition.[7]

Assessment by a Neurologist

Specific aspects of a patient's health exist that are normally examined by neurologists to determine the efficiency and working order of the CNS. The intent of a neurologist is to assess a patient suffering from this disorder by checking[8]:

- memory and cognition
- language and speech
- reflexes
- nerves in the neck and head
- overall balance and posture
- muscle strength and restrictive movement

Common Tests Performed by a Neurologist

In order to determine the exact nature of pain and the nature of the medical condition, neurologists will examine motley areas of the peripheral nervous system as well as the CNS. The examination and evaluation is based on several diagnostic tests, some of which help present a visual impression of a patient's brain. These tests also help to spot malfunctioning nerves and muscles. The most frequent diagnostic tests include[9]:

- MRI (magnetic resonance imaging)
- CAT scan (computed axial tomography)
- EMG (electromyography)
- EEG (electroencephalography)

These diagnostic procedures are conducted using state-of-the-art medical equipment and are overseen by the neurologist.

Treatment Plan Provided by a Neurologist

With the test results, the neurologist will be on a better locus to recommend the most effective treatment plan so that the patient can find relief from specific symptoms. Neurologists normally recommend a continuous treatment scheme with frequent checkups and are responsible for observing the by and large progress of patients. It is common for neurologists to advocate a combination therapy that includes medical treatments, medication, exercise, and physical therapy. The most commonly recommended neurological treatments for FM are[10]:

- pain medications, including antiepileptic drugs (AED), antidepressants, anti-inflammatory pain killers, sleep aids, and muscle relaxants
- trigger point injections (TPI) administered to suppress pain emanating from a tender point
- nerve blocks, either a therapeutic nerve block used mainly to treat painful conditions and relying on the use of a local anesthetic, or a preemptive nerve block used to throttle subsequent pain
- alternative therapies, such as swimming, meditation, and yoga, to fight stress and achieve sound sleep

ROLES OF OTHER PHYSICIANS IN FIBROMYALGIA

Internists, family medical practitioners, and psychologists can treat depression, anxiety, and sleeping disorders. These three symptoms require the use of medication and changes in lifestyle. The scopic problem begins when an individual is faced with FM-related pain. This type of pain can subsist in a precise area of the body, such as the back of the neck, or can cause widespread aching across the entire body. The specific areas that cause pain are known as trigger points. These areas can feel tired or overworked even when an individual has not been performing any physical exercise or workouts. The patient can experience twitching muscles or experience persistent aching along with a stabbing pain. Patients with FM can experience pain around their hips, along the joints in their neck, back, and shoulders. This throbbing and unrelenting pain can make it difficult for patients to lead a normal life. Whatever the type or degree of pain, it can be treated by physicians and medical practitioners using a variety of methods.[11]

DIAGNOSIS OF FM BY PHYSICIANS

A physician plays a critical role in diagnosing the various symptoms and drawing a conclusion for a treatment path. *Diagnosis* should be done by a qualified physician, as most of the symptoms of FM exist in other medical conditions as well. It is important for the physician to rule out every other medical condition prior to articulating the FM diagnosis.

The physician can also recommend specific laboratory tests to conduct, including[12]:

- blood tests, particularly the complete blood count (CBC) to study the red and white cells, hemoglobin, and platelets
- kidney and liver tests to check the blood chemistry
- thyroid tests to identify an underactive or overactive thyroid

Apart from these, a physician will also conduct several other tests to check the red blood cell sedimentation rate, to test for the rheumatoid factor, and to scan for anti-CCP antibodies. During the examination process, a physician will try to derive as much information as possible by[13]:

- checking the patient's body for widespread pain
- asking the patient about fatigue and lack of sleep
- evaluating stress levels
- identifying and evaluating the various trigger points
- conducting tests for depression

The physician, while determining the diagnosis, will take into account the following criteria[14]:

- pain is present in the body or a specific part of the body for a minimum of three months
- pain is widespread and in all quadrants of the body
- tests and other examinations indicate that the patient is not suffering from any other disease with similar symptoms

In retrospect, the best way to go about diagnosis is by conducting a thorough physical examination of the patient followed by identification and discourse of the various symptoms, as this will help the doctor to determine whether or not the symptoms are related to FM. For example, during the physical examination the physician may pinpoint the tender points, but only when the doctor and patient deliberate on the nature and intensity of the pain can a proper diagnosis and treatment plan be attained.[15]

8

PREVENTION IS THE KEY

Ben Franklin once said, "An ounce of prevention is worth a pound of cure," and that holds true for all types of medical conditions, including FM. Even in the medical orb, doctors and other practitioners admit that prevention is preferable to treatment. The oath taken by graduating doctors ensconces a similar phrase: "I will prevent disease whenever I can, for prevention is preferable to cure." The big question then becomes: Why is prevention of a medical condition such as FM so meaningful? To understand its significance, it is necessary to understand what prevention is and how it is entwined with everyday life.[1]

LIFESTYLE AND ITS ROLE IN THE PREVENTION OF FIBROMYALGIA

Fibromyalgia pain and symptoms can be reduced through a lifestyle change. It is a challenge, but it is possible. The patient must keep in mind that action is power. He or she must be aware that medications alone are not enough to treat FM. Lifestyle changes are necessary and essential for the treatment of symptoms and for pain relief. The person affected with FM must learn to be proactive. Good sleep is associated with a good lifestyle, but without invigorating rest the patient cannot progress in the treatment of FM. Insomnia, which is common in FM patients, must be uprooted. A good diet is necessary; the patient must avoid foods that trigger or worsen the symptoms. To minimize the pain and fatigue, the patient must make lifestyle adjustments.[2]

Education about the disease is likewise necessary. The FM sufferer can request assistance from medical professionals, support groups, and other FM patients. Doctors and other medical professionals, such as physical therapists and nutritionists, can advise patients on how to best approach the treatment and relief of symptoms. These authorities can help patients understand the importance of taking care of themselves. They can offer tips such as keeping warm as soon as they begin to feel cold or during periods of chronic pain.[3]

The patient must learn constructive mechanics for standing, sitting, and other positions. He must keep active, taking into consideration personal limitations, avoiding excessive exercise, and, most importantly, choosing the exercises that are appropriate to active symptoms. Exercise plays a vital role in the treatment of FM. The patient should manage a healthy, active life, and exercise, such as walking or water exercise, is essential for the treatment of this disease. Patients must enter an exercise program that meets their specific individual needs, focusing on muscle functionality and tone. Fibromyalgia patients consult their doctors before beginning any exercise routine so that the doctor can review medical records and conduct an examination, taking into consideration the factors that impact the disease. Although pain and fatigue sometimes hinder the patient's ability to effectuate aerobics, every effort must be made to exercise. The patient must dedicate time for daily exercise. Twenty to thirty minutes per day almost every day is recommended. A new exercise routine must be started bit by bit, and the activity or exertion level must develop slowly too. The patient should begin with a few minutes of exercise per day and build up until reaching the ideal length of time. Before and after exercising, stretching is urged. Stretching with breathing is important, and after exercising, a hot bath or shower is laudatory.[4]

REST AND ITS ROLE IN THE PREVENTION OF FIBROMYALGIA

The patients must learn their limits, such as when they need to rest and when they can partake in active situations. Patients must pace daytime activities. They must practice relaxation before bedtime to help maximize sleep. A hot bath, hot water bottles, or heated blanket are examples of things that can be included in the bedtime routine to help induce sleep. The patient must create the necessary environment to lead the body to a restorative snooze. In the case of insomnia, the patient should consider meditation. Fatigue and other aggravating symptoms can lead patients into immobility. Patients become unable to carry out daily routines, and the chronic pain hinders daily chores and responsibilities at home, at work, and at school. The patient, sometimes due to invalidity, becomes unable to work and needs financial support.[5]

Fibromyalgia patients typically have poor sleep quality, and this must be taken care of. The pain worsens the sleep and vice versa. The patient must take steps to tweak their sleep quality level[6]:

- Contrive and strictly follow a sleep schedule. Go to bed every night and rise every morning at the same time.
- The room temperature must be cool enough to sleep comfortably. A warm room spoils the quality of sleep.
- Caffeine, including products such as coffee, chocolate, tea, and colas, must be avoided beginning in the early evening. Alcohol, too, must be eliminated from the diet. Some people say alcohol is necessary for prompting sleep, but that is not true, and in fact it has the opposite effect.
- Exercise is essential to a good night's sleep. Exercise should not be done in the evening because it makes it difficult to fall asleep.
- Napping during the day must be avoided as it takes away the tranquility of nighttime sleep. The bedroom must be comfortable to promote a good sleep. Ironically, the slow hum of a fan can create a good sensation for sleep.
- To relax at bedtime, the patient can listen to soft music before falling asleep. Reading a good book is also recommended to provoke the relaxation need to improve sleep quality.
- Creating and following a comfortable bedtime routine every night will help the patient to have a good night's rest.

A sleep routine must be established to get rid of fatigue. Sleep disturbance must be treated adequately to avoid pain. The patient, with the help of family members, must find the covetable conditions to produce good sleep quality. Without a normal sleep cycle, the symptoms, such as pain and fatigue, don't wane; on the contrary, the sufferer feels even worse from day to day without restorative sleep. It is also recommended, besides avoiding alcohol and caffeine, that the patient not imbibe any liquids before going to bed to avoid the need to wake and go to the bathroom during the night. To have good sleep, physicians recommend that the patient remain calm during the evening and night (about six hours before going to bed). If the FM patient follows these guidelines, he or she will have a significant improvement in overall health, and will be able to manage a normal life without pain. This will lead to keeping an active daily life and to a high level of self-esteem.[7]

SCOPE OF PREVENTION IN MEDICAL SCIENCE

In medical terms, prevention or preventive actions are directed toward avoidance of specific medical conditions, illnesses, disorders, or diseases. The concept of prevention revolves around the promotion of the overall health of people of different gender and age sets in such a way that their need for primary, secondary, or tertiary health care is exceedingly reduced.[8]

The scope of prevention in a medical sense relates to averting any type of development of a pathological state or a physical condition that has been caused by a disease or disorder. At the same time, there is a broader perspective of prevention as well, and it includes seizing various measures, including definitive therapy for limiting the progression of any disease at any given stage.[9]

The stage at which a disease or medical condition is prevented from occurring is known as primary prevention, and secondary prevention is applied to bar the disease or medical condition from becoming worse. Prevention of a medical condition such as FM includes a set of actions that are geared toward reducing or eliminating the onset of the medical condition, causes of a disease, complications that surface from the disorder, and finally the recurrence of the medical condition.[10]

The set of actions required varies from one medical condition to another and is also dependent on the medical history of the individual patient, the existing medications, and the stage of the disease. A set of actions will usually consist of three processes[11]:

- Nursing action includes risk assessment of the medical condition with or without conducting tests.
- Application includes applying prescribed measures for prevention at the dawning of disease or symptoms and can include immunization and educating the patient regarding the medical condition.
- Early diagnosis is conducted by a medical professional or family physician and includes proper diagnosis of the disease, symptoms, and rehabilitation outlook.

NEED AND SIGNIFICANCE OF PREVENTIVE CARE

There is an inherent need for applying prevention tactics in the daily lives of people around the world as it will help them lead better and healthier lives. There is a penury of *primary prevention* tactics that should be part of everyday life, and this includes how and where the patients live, work, learn, and play. Even though medical professionals realize the need and significance of primary prevention for medical conditions including FM, more often than not they end up facing several barriers. These barriers stop doctors from helping patients effectively prevent diseases or disorders. The obstacles can be purely educational in nature or can include behavioral, economic, and cultural factors. Some of the most common include mass ignorance, lack of choice, and cultural pressures.[12]

Unfamiliarity or lack of knowledge related to the risk associated with a medical condition is one of the ramparts of prevention. Lack of knowledge often leads to a high-risk behavior among people, which can be one of the primary causes for disorders or diseases. Many times, people choose to ignore or disregard the preventive advice provided to them by nursing professionals or family physicians, such as overmedication.[13]

Lack of choice is another barrier in the path of preventive care. For example, a lack of funds or poor finances may force patients to deny themselves preventive care to avoid medical fees. Absence of choice can also include unavailability of proper health care services within a reasonable distance.[14]

Cultural or societal pressure normally affects teenagers and young people more than the elderly. Such pressure often induces young people to display high-risk behaviors, which in the long run can be detrimental to the vigor of those individuals. In such cases, a serious injury or medical condition can arise before de rigueur steps of prevention can be taken. In more ways than one, this pressure is also connected to ignorance or lack of knowledge.[15]

Preventive care can take place on three different stratums: national, local, and personal. Care on a national level takes place through hospitals and clinics supported by the government and include prevention tactics as well as the dissemination of information using mass media platforms such as newspapers and television. On a local level, preventive care is implemented by the local government and includes both prevention tactics and health education. On a personal level, each individual needs to include certain practices in day-to-day life, including the decisions made regarding lifestyle choices. Individuals can also consult a family physician from time to time regarding specific ailments in order to foil existing medical conditions. Prevention is all about risk reduction, and this process can be followed for FM and the like.[16]

Fibromyalgia is a medical condition or disorder with principal symptoms of fatigue and muscle pain. People suffering from FM will experience tender points in various parts of their body. The most common tender points occur in and around the shoulders, neck, hips, back, legs, and arms. These points become so tender that they hurt or ache even with the slightest pressure. Some of the other symptoms that people with FM may experience include headache, trouble sleeping, painful menstrual periods, morning stiffness, problems with memory and concentration, and numbness or tingling sensations in the hands and feet.[17]

There is a high probability that people suffering from FM may experience multiple chronic or severe pain conditions. Although there are no official studies to show how and why FM occurs, they are linked to a variety of events that are recognized as likely causes. These include stressful events, repetitive injury, long spells of illness and certain diseases, and traumatic incidents including car accidents.[18]

PREVENTIVE CARE FOR FIBROMYALGIA

The big question is: Can FM be prevented? Yes, it can be prevented if the necessary steps are taken. Prevention can take place only when the root cause is identified. Since lack of sleep, physical and emotional stress, taxing workload, and erratic lifestyle and habits are considered as some of the critical factors, this is where prevention needs to launch. Each of the contributing factors needs to be dealt with separately, and addressing these issues can help prevent the onset of FM. The factors are fatigue, stress, and lack of sleep.[19]

Fatigue must be prevented or relieved. The two best ways of preventing fatigue are by increasing exercise and avoiding caffeine and alcohol. Most people would think that exercise would increase tiredness, so how can it be that it actually prevents fatigue? The fact is that a proper exercise regimen, if followed daily under the guidance of a professional instructor, can be one of the best ways to boost physical capacity (i.e., by way of fitness and weight loss). In the long run, regular exercise, such as a thirty-minute walk, can be quite therapeutic and can increase overall well-being. Other suggested workouts include moderate-intensity exercises, cycling, swimming, and aerobics. Fibromyalgia patients should avoid caffeine and alcohol because these are not only poison for the body but are known forestallers of proper sleep. Caffeine and alcohol deprive people of their recommended eight hours of sleep, and the next morning they tend to wake up tired. Eschewing caffeine and alcohol before bedtime can help prevent tiredness in the morning.[20]

Stress can be considered a nemesis of the modern age, and anyone can be prone to it at various junctures of life. Some people are prone to work stress while others suffer from stress caused by specific incidents, such as accidents, fear, financial issues, and even personal or home issues. If the excess stress can be avoided, then it will be easier to prevent FM to a great extent. One of the most common ways of thwarting stress-induced FM is relaxation therapy. It plays a critical role in the prevention of FM and can be done at home or at venues that offer maximum relaxation through various therapies. Relaxation techniques can help in reducing various beacons of stress by lowering blood pressure, slowing down the heart rate, increasing proper blood flow to major arteries and muscles, reducing overall activity of various stress hormones, slowing the breathing rate, offsetting chronic pain and muscle tension, reducing fatigue, improving mood and concentration, and dropping frustration and anger.[21]

There are several different types of relaxation techniques that can be followed to reduce stress and prevent FM. These include deep-breath-

ing meditation, progressive muscle relaxation exercises, body scan meditation, mindfulness meditation, visualization meditation for peace and
relaxation, yoga exercises, and tai chi.[22]

The third and probably one of the most important factors causing
FM is lack of sleep. Sleep deprivation also contributes to other factors
such as stress, anxiety, and fatigue. The best way to fight this is to follow
a sleeping cycle and get better sleep. There are many different ways of
preventing sleep deprivation or insomnia[23]:

- Train the body to wake up at the same time every day.
- Eliminate caffeine, nicotine, and alcohol as they hamper sound
  sleep.
- Reduce or eliminate napping as it can affect the quality of sleep at
  night.
- Exercise regularly to help improve the overall quality of sleep.
- Avoid eating or drinking fluids before bedtime as it can cause
  instabilities in sleep.
- Reduce all type of activities in bed except sleeping, such as mak-
  ing phone calls, working on a laptop, or playing games.
- Create a comfortable sleeping environment conducive to good
  quality sleep, including a comfortable bed and mattress, dim light-
  ing, and low noise.
- It is essential to leave all worries and thoughts behind as they can
  keep the brain working and disturb sleep.
- Participate in cognitive therapy to identify the root causes of insomnia and eliminate them.
- Use meditation or relaxation therapy techniques prior to sleep.
- Listening to soft music can be extremely helpful in falling asleep.

Last but not least, good sleep can work wonders for the mind and
body. Sleep is not only fundamental for the brain and nervous system to
function properly but also to ensure every part of the body, including
muscles, is relaxed. Life is not easy for patients suffering from nervous
system disorders and FM, but there are ways to whisk the pain away.
One can reduce the overall impact of nervous system disorders by preventing FM. "Health is wealth," and with age, health can be severely
affected. The bottom line is that by pursuing a healthy lifestyle encom-
passing a well-balanced diet, proper exercises, less stress, and sufficient

sleep, people can actually reduce the risk of FM and thus circumvent their overall health risk and increase well-being in toto.[24]

HOW CAN PREVENTION IMPROVE THE QUALITY OF LIFE FOR FM PATIENTS?

Can the prevention of FM or any of its symptoms help improve the quality of life for patients suffering from other nervous system disorders? Yes, because FM is a disorder that is allied to the malfunctioning of the central nervous system (CNS). If a person is already suffering from a nervous system disorder such as *Parkinson's* disease, multiple sclerosis, or *Alzheimer's*, then the symptoms of FM can actually exacerbate the disorder. For example, a person suffering from Alzheimer's will experience nuisances with memory and concentration, and symptoms of FM, including anxiousness and depression, can worsen the existing medical condition. Hence, prevention of FM is important for those already suffering from some other ilk of nervous system disorder.[25]

PREVENTION OF FIBROMYALGIA FOR OVERALL WELL-BEING

It is indeed true that prevention of FM will not only reduce the intensity of various nervous system conditions but will also ensure people enjoy overall well-being and a healthy life. The most important thing that people need to realize is that the nervous system itself is responsible for the sentiment of well-being. A disorder in the nervous system can affect consciousness and the ability to think and perceive; to focus or concentrate to remember (affecting both short-term and long-term memory); to solve problems; to yield decisions; to create, plan, and execute; to learn, read, and write; and to express emotions or communicate.[26]

If a specific constituent of the nervous system is impaired, then it can affect various parts of the body and the activities related to it. What can people suffering from various nervous system disorders do? How can people clutch prosperity by preventing FM? When people work toward putting a stop to the occurrence of FM then they can experience a feeling of restfulness, the absence of pain, muscles that work in coordination, and an uplifted mood. This might sound simple, but to patients who suffer from chronic FM pain, the relief of these symptoms is just that—relief.[27]

Tiredness or fatigue can be quite threatening to someone suffering from nervous system disorders. Tiredness caused by prolonged exercise can lead to central nervous system fatigue, while bleariness arising out of a sleep disorder can lead to chronic fatigue syndrome. This can be completely avoided by following sleep routines, sleeping well, exercising in a balanced way, meditating, and practicing relaxation therapies. When fatigue is eliminated, the patient will be one step closer to averting FM, and the absence of this condition will ensure better overall health in people already suffering from neurological conditions.[28]

Prevention of FM will make certain that people do not suffer from tender point pain and burning pain. Pain can sometimes be quite irritating and can be utterly exhausting and overwhelming as well. Pain has the ability to take away peace of mind, which in turn will affect the overall well-being of patients. Proper exercises and ways of relaxing the muscles can have an acquiescent effect on the body and provide necessary relief from pain.[29]

Fibromyalgia can cause widespread pain in different muscles or muscle groups. Symptoms such as cramping, weakness, muscle knots, and itchy muscles are fairly common in FM, and the increase in their force can be disadvantageous for patients suffering from nervous system disorders. Nervous system disorders such as autoimmune disorders (i.e., Isaac syndrome), Lou Gehrig's disease, and spinal muscular atrophy affect muscles in the body, and the prevention of FM will ensure that those muscles do not degenerate any further.[30]

The type of mood people have can affect their behavior and decision making. The primary causes of extreme mood swings are neurotransmitters and hormones. That said, clients suffering from nervous system disorders such as multiple sclerosis will experience rash mood changes. In such a scenario, FM symptoms will only augment mood sensitivity in patients. A nifty way to prevent FM or any of its symptoms from flaring up is to practice mood therapy. The further people are from depression and anxiety, the better their mental and mood health will be. Mood therapies, for example, meditation, yoga, and cognitive-behavioral therapies, can be highly productive in such a scenario. [31]

III

Common Ways of Coping

ALTERNATIVE THERAPIES

What could be better than natural treatments? That is what herbal treatments are all about—helping people find a natural substitute for the treatment of FM. Fibromyalgia is not a phantom disorder that cannot be treated, but there are two slants toward successful treatment: traditional treatment and herbal treatment. Traditional alimentation includes medications prescribed by doctors and can involve everything from muscle pain medications such as cyclobenzaprine and *narcotic analgesics*.[1]

Different symptoms of FM have to be treated separately, and this means most patients are counselled on a long list of medications. When this happens, there is always a possibility or risk of one medication reacting with another. Herbal therapy is an integral part of alternative tactics for FM. This treatment also follows a similar path as traditional treatment in that different herbs and therapies are prearranged for different signs related to this disorder. The advantage that herbal treatment has over traditional treatment is that there are no side effects, nor do herbs react with any other form of treatment.[2]

TENS

Transcutaneous electrical nerve stimulation (TENS) therapy delivers electric impulses in painful areas, stimulating the nerve tissues to release pain-fighting chemicals. TENS is used in the assuagement of FM and other diseases such as arthritis. TENS therapy is efficient in relieving pain and is performed in conjunction with other therapies, such as heat or cold therapy or massage. A professional therapist performs TENS therapy. The treatment session lasts about one hour. It is so painless that many fall asleep during the procedure. The patient can buy a TENS device and perform this therapy at home.[3]

HERBAL OPTIONS

There are several different herbal remedy options available for treatment of FM, and these treatments vary according to the type of symptoms, nature of symptoms, intensity of symptoms, and how long the symptoms have existed.[4]

Muscle and Other Pain. One of the most common and easily decipherable symptoms of FM is muscle pain and tenderness in various parts of the body. Pain can be unremitting and throbbing or can vary from low to high intensity. Natural remedies can prove to be extremely effective in helping reduce the pain, and this includes the application or oral consumption of a variety of herbs. Ginger extract has been in use for centuries to halt inflammation and joint pain. Capsaicin is used for pain management and is derived from spicy hot cayenne peppers. It can be consumed in raw or powdered form or can be applied in the form of a topical cream.[5]

Turmeric is considered a splendid herbal remedy because of its variety of healing properties. Turmeric has the ability to reduce inflammation, heartburn, and pain caused by arthritis or other joint pain. Devil's Claw is a native South African shrub that has the ability to provide relief from neck, shoulder, and low back impediments and is often prescribed as an anti-inflammatory pain medication. In addition, menthol and camphor are considered two of the best herbal fillips for the treatment of neck pain occurring in FM. Menthol and camphor can also provide relief from joint or muscle ache and are normally used in the form of essential oils, creams, and gels. Some of the other herbs used for making a stand against FM pain and muscle cramps include St. John's wort and valerian root.[6]

Anxiety and Depression. Anxiety and depression can happen to anyone, but when they appear with other symptoms of FM they can disturb a person's everyday activities. The best way to fight anxiety and depression is by taking the herbal course. Remedies available include chamomile, green tea, lemon balm, and St. John's wort. Chamomile tea is considered the number-one herbal remedy for thumping anxiety and other related symptoms of stress and FM. Green tea is one of the healthiest herbal foods. It not only helps subdue anxiety but also increases concentration and alertness, curbs blood pressure, and stabilizes heart rate. Lemon balm has a long history of use and is used primarily for reducing stress and anxiety. The therapeutic effects also help achieve sound sleep. Moreover, St. John's wort is considered an effective herbal contrivance for treating mild to moderate cases of depression.[7]

Insomnia and Fatigue. Lack of sleep is one of the most irritating and exhausting symptoms of FM. In fact, privation of sound sleep is one of the causes of fatigue, which is another symptom of FM. Herbal remedies can not only treat insomnia and fatigue effectively but also ensure the recovery is permanent. Some of the commonly used herbs include valerian, California poppy, and passionflower. Valerian is an herbal remedy used for the treatment of sleep disorders in patients anguishing from FM. Valerian is used in the form of extract and essential oils and can be used for the treatment of other symptoms such as chronic fatigue, depression, and anxiety. Another extremely effective herbal remedy, California poppy, promotes relaxation. It is used for treating sleep issues such as insomnia, nervous agitation, bladder problems such as frequent urination, and aches, among other symptoms. Passionflower is a powerful yet soothing herb often ordered for patients suffering from several symptoms of FM, such as insomnia and anxiety. Passionflower is offered in the form of tea, tincture, liquid extract, and infusion. With intact sleep cycles, fatigue disappears on its own, but if tiredness continues to persist, then certain herbs can be used. These herbs include Siberian ginseng, licorice root, sea kelp, Indian ginseng or Withania, Schizandra, and Astragalus, among others. One of the salient aspects of alternative treatment of FM is that patients can leverage the various remedies available in order to facilitate speedy recovery.[8]

THE MAGIC OF MASSAGE THERAPY FOR FIBROMYALGIA

Massage therapy is recommended for mild pain. A massage with mild pressure brings good results. The patient's physician can recommend a good therapist who can perform the pain-relieving massage. A professional therapist must be licensed. Massage does not cure FM but it is very helpful for reducing symptoms. Massage stimulates endorphin production. With good massage therapy the patient can reduce the use of medication, but the relief is temporary, lasting about six months. Although massage is usually performed by a massage therapist, it can also be performed by the patient's partner or a friend. The patient can also use a mechanical massager, but he must abide by precautions with the high cycle so as to not redouble the pain. When the massage is not performed by a professional therapist, precautions must be taken. As with all therapies, massage therapy is not adequate for everyone. Massage is not recommended for a person with chronic migraines, a patient who has had brain surgery, a patient with a family history of epilepsy and seizures, pregnant women, and patients with cardiac pacemakers or other implanted devices.[9]

Can massage therapy really work for FM patients? The truth is that it can do wonders. Fibromyalgia is a chronic musculoskeletal condition in which the symptoms revolve around muscles, pain, insomnia, and fatigue. The role that massage therapy plays is that of providing relaxation and solace from such symptoms. It is best to find professional massage therapists and body workers who have the experience of working with patients suffering from FM and chronic fatigue syndrome. So how does massage therapy really work? Are there any specific techniques that are used? Professional massage therapists use different techniques to reduce the discomfort and pain associated with FM. Massage is a method of achieving relaxation, and it acts toward the following[10]:

- encouraging circulation in different muscles
- increasing the flow of important nutrients entailed by the body
- reducing increased heart rate
- relegating pain
- accruing the body's ability to fight pain
- reducing aches in joints to increase the range of motion

• relaxing mind, body, and muscles

There are a variety of effective techniques used by body workers and physical therapists for FM patients.

Oxygen Massage Therapy. The mission of this type of relaxing massage is to enable oxygenation. This is a therapeutic massage technique that focuses on deep tissue healing, relieving muscle cramps and pain, and injury rehabilitation. This therapy helps by "unbolting" the muscles and joints that have been locked in a spasm. At the same time, it also provides relief to those patients suffering from severe neck pain and experiencing tightness in their lower back region. [11]

Lumbar Massage Therapy. Lumbar massage therapy, as the name suggests, rivets on providing relief from lower back pain and is used most often as an effective adjunct for different types of lower back conundrums. This massage therapy has three major benefits for FM patients. Lumbar massage helps in enriching overall blood circulation, and this helps muscles to recover from pain, soreness, and cramps. The massage therapy relaxes different muscles in the body in such a way that the range of motion of muscles improves significantly. Relaxed muscles help fight insomnia issues as well. The massage causes endorphin levels to increase. Endorphins are chemicals ceded by the body to ensure the proper management of chronic pain. [12]

Neuromuscular Massage Therapy (NMT). Neuromuscular massage therapy focuses on applying different levels of concentrated pressure specifically on areas of the body deteriorating from muscle spasm. Massage therapists apply pressure using their knuckles, fingers, or elbows. There are several benefits of this type of kneading for FM patients. Lumbar massage helps relieve tension and pain in and around the shoulder and neck. Massage in the upper back area helps vitiate pain caused by migraine. This therapy technique helps in releasing serotonin and dopamine, which are "feel good" compounds manufactured naturally by the body. The release of such chemicals helps in pain management, prevents depression and anxiety, and improves sleep. [13]

Transcranial Magnetic Stimulation. Transcranial magnetic stimulation is approved by the FDA and is effective in pain relief. The nerve cells are stimulated by electrical current, bringing pain relief. The sequence takes about thirty minutes. [14]

Chiropractic Therapy. Chiropractors are not medical doctors but are competent and licensed to perform procedures related to the spine, such as realignments. The professional must take care to execute the procedure gently.[15]

Positional Release Therapy. Osteopathic physicians normally practice this therapy. It is a specialized technique that is considered a part of modern-day massage therapy for the eradication of FM symptoms. There are different types of techniques employed in this therapy, and the most common among them are the strain counterstrain (SCS) technique and the muscle energy technique. These practices are used for the treatment of protective muscle spasms in the human body. The system involves locating tender points in the body such as muscles, tendons, ligaments, and joints. Once the tender point is located, then the rest of the patient's body is refocused away from the specific area with tenderness toward a position that is of pronounced comfort. The tender points normally treated through this procedure include the following[16]:

- biceps
- the hip flexor
- the intercostal muscles between the ribs
- the trapezius in the upper back and neck
- plantar fascia (the tissues and muscles of the feet)
- lumbar area (muscles of the back)
- cervical and scapular (muscles of the head and neck)
- the tibialis posterior (leg muscle)
- patellar tendon (a ligament in the knee)
- iliotibial band (the IT band that connects the hip and the knee)

Swedish Massage Technique. Swedish massage is recommended for patients of FM as it is different from regular massage techniques. The techniques focus on applying deep pressure on different parts of the body to enhance the liberation of metabolic waste such as uric and lactic acid from muscle tissues and also to ensure superior oxygenation of blood. This massage therapy helps to impede stiffness and pain in joints, helps to relieve physical and emotional stress, and induces sound sleep. There are five different types of Swedish massage techniques used for FM patients:

- Effleurage is a gliding or sliding massage technique that focuses on relieving tension and knots in the muscles.
- Friction caused by rubbing produces heat and causes the muscle to relax.
- Petrissage involves the kneading of muscles and leads to deep massage penetration.
- Vibration uses a back and forth action of the heel of therapist's hands or fingertips over the patient's skin to help loosen muscles.
- Rhythmic tapping or tapotement uses a fist made of cupped hands, and this technique helps to loosen and relax various muscles of the body.[17]

Reflexology Massage Therapy. Reflexology is a massage therapy of the feet and has been in use since ancient China. It uses the philosophy that the human feet contain several energy channels known as meridian points. When these points are stimulated, they promote relaxation and healing. Corresponding to reflexology theory, each point on the foot relates to a specific organ or area in the human body. The stimulation of each point can effectively improve or heal the organ or the part of the body it corresponds to. Hence, reflexology massage is often regarded as a complete body massage. Reflexology massage technique helps to vanquish stress, increase energy flow, incite the digestive system, reduce pain, provide sound sleep, and increment blood circulation. The reflexology massage technique involves pressure harnessed with the thumb, or finger walking. This simply means that a professional reflexologist will stammer their thumb or finger over different points on the feet while applying pressure to get the desired outcome.[18]

Reflexology demonstrates four primary effects:

- amelioration of various symptoms or bringing about positive tunings in the functioning of different organs in the body
- impacts on the functioning of specific organs such as an increase of blood flow to the intestines or kidney
- creation of a relaxation effect that helps ebb anxiety and decrease blood pressure
- aids in reducing a variety of pain, including neck pain, chest pain, back pain, and pain from osteoarthritis[19]

Trigger Point Therapy. This therapy is often considered one of the best massage therapies for FM. Trigger point therapy, as the name indicates, is a type of massage therapy that focuses on specific areas within a muscle tissue responsible for triggering pain in other parts of the body. Trigger points are ultimately painful spots situated in muscle fiber bands, and patients suffering from FM normally have more trigger points as compared to people with other painful conditions. How does it work? If an FM patient has a point on the back of the neck that is bringing on pain in the whole lumbar region, then the massage therapist will focus on affording relief to the neck pain or the trigger point. The trigger points are deactivated using finger pressure, and the denouement is always positive and relaxing and leads to the proper management of FM pain.[20]

Acupuncture for Fibromyalgia. Acupuncture (commonly confused with acupressure) has been known to bring about considerable pain relief. It must be performed by a medical doctor, osteopathic physician, or nurse practitioner. The application of pins stimulates the production of endorphins (pain-fighting chemicals in the brain), which brings pain relief. The result is temporary.[21]

There are a variety of alternative treatments, but among FM patients, the usefulness of acupuncture is probably the least well known. It is important to first understand what acupuncture really is. Acupuncture is an alternative treatment that has existed in Traditional Chinese Medicine (TCM) for centuries. Traditional acupuncture, a pattern of noninvasive therapy, is actually considered to be one of the most effective methods of reducing FM symptoms. The philosophy behind this healing emphasizes that the entire human body consists of energy, also known as chi or qi energy, and is the vital cogency of life. This energy flows through meridians. It is believed that some of the symptoms of FM such as pain, insomnia, and tiredness occur when an imbalance is created in the flow of qi energy. Acupuncture helps by reinstating the balance and thus restores a proper flow of qi energy, which provides relief from pain and insomnia.[22]

Fibromyalgia corresponds to abnormalities in the central pain-processing unit of the brain. The abnormality releases neurotransmitters such as noradrenaline and serotonin, which lowers the pain threshold in patients. So how can acupuncture help in such a scenario? Acupuncture is known to stimulate various points in the human body that further stimulate the nervous system. This process of stimulation helps in releasing neurochemical messenger molecules. The emission of molecules initiates a biochemical change that influences the homeostatic mechanism of the human body. The chemicals promote physical as well as emotional well-being. One of the important things to understand here is that not all acupuncture points can be stimulated to reduce pain. There are specific points that affect separate areas of the body, especially the zone that controls pain management. Hence, the acupuncture needs to be run by a professional and experienced acupuncturist only.[23]

Traditionally, this process uses fine, thin needles, which are inserted into various pressure points spanning the body. The insertion of a needle fuels the pressure points or meridians to provide relief from a variety of pain, including muscle pain, joint pain, lower back pain, and migraine. The thought of piercing needles can sound daunting, but professional acupuncturists take care in how they are inserted. The needles are sterilized prior to and after each insertion.[24]

Acupuncture helps patients to find relief from pain orchestrated by FM, and it achieves this by[25]:

- stimulating the nerves situated in various muscles and tissues throughout the body. This stimulation causes the release of endorphins, which further helps in changing the pain processing in the human brain and spinal cord.
- altering a patient's brain chemistry, which helps in increasing endorphins as well as neuropeptide Y levels and at the same time abating serotonin levels.
- promoting the release of immunomodulatory and vascular factors, which plays an important role in reducing inflammation.
- improving upon existing and overall joint mobility and muscle stiffness, and it achieves this by increasing local microcirculation.

Acupuncture can also be accomplished along with other traditional Chinese medical treatments such as moxibustion or the application of heat and laser light, depending on the patient's condition.

Hot and Cold for Fibromyalgia. A common alternative treatment used by medical professionals to provide relief from FM symptoms is the hot and cold method. It is an effective alternate treatment for tender points, but it has to be applied carefully as some FM sufferers may have increased sensitivity to heat or cold. Hence, the type of treatment varies from one patient to the next.[26]

Hydrotherapy, performed in a pool, can relieve pain and improve sleep quality. Exercises such as warmups, stretching, aerobics, and relaxation movements are primed in water. The results of hydrotherapy are better than conventional physical therapy. The patient can perform water walking (walking around the pool). Water therapy brings pain relief. Care must be taken in hot water because it can enflame the symptoms if the temperature is too high. Use of a hot tub can be precarious and should not be used if the patient is alone.[27]

Heat Therapy. Heat therapy is the preferred therapy for body pain as it has consistently shown to have the most positive results. An expert performs this therapy using heat to increase blood flow in the aching area to help the healing process. The heat helps but does not eliminate pain. It is an appropriate therapy for cases of chronic pain. The heat causes the muscles to relax and convalesces circulation. Hot baths and massage therapy are effective for providing pain relief. The patient can use heat therapy with gel packs at home. It is recommended that the patient use care with regard to the temperature. Too much heat can exacerbate symptoms rather than relieve them.[28]

Heat therapy is considered to be strong in the treatment of FM symptoms. There are different methods that can be used and are known to provide gains, such as[29]:

- increased blood flow
- increased blood vessel dilation
- increased metabolic rate
- significant reduction of pain in and around tender points
- increased soft tissue extensibility
- removal of wastes and toxins
- decreased joint stiffness by increasing flexibility of the connective tissue
- decreased muscle and pain spasm
- reduced inflammation caused by muscle spasms, strain or sprain, and arthritis
- relief from chronic headache and stress
- restful sleep

There are several different types of heat therapies, including heat pads or warm baths. Heating pads or wraps target specific areas, particularly tender points. Warm baths, jacuzzis, spas, or hot water tubs are considered an excellent heat therapy for mitigating back pain caused by FM. A hot bath also encourages restful sleep. [30]

Cold therapy, also called cryotherapy, uses cold instead of heat to treat pain and inflammation. This therapy is not recommended for cold-sensitive patients. The patient can do this at home with gel packs, for example. The result is temporary; the pain relief lasts about seven hours. [31]

Heat and cold therapy, hydrotherapy, and massage can be performed in combination. For example, a patient can undergo a mild massage in combination with heat or cold therapy. The result is great and provides the necessary respite. [32]

Homeopathy. This brings pain relief to the tender points. The use of herbs is efficient in the treatment of many diseases, including FM. Homeopathy is performed by a homoeopath. [33]

Surgery for Fibromyalgia. Fibromyalgia can be perceived as a pain-amplifying condition, yet surgery is always the last option. It is a known fact that trigger points or tender points cannot be surgically removed, but specific neck, lower back, or neurological disorders associated with FM can be surgically rectified. When is surgery possible for FM patients? Surgery is promising only in certain circumstances [34]:

- when a neck injury of a patient suffering from FM has led to the creation of a pain trigger point
- when there is too much pressure on the spinal cord or nerve roots giving rise to severe pain, numbness in hands or legs, and loss of bowel control
- when an FM patient is suffering from knee pain caused by arthritis or similar medical conditions
- when a pinched nerve in the leg causes extreme leg pain
- when motor nerves have been damaged, causing muscle twitching
- when damage has been caused in the sensory nerves causing the FM patient to experience extreme pain, numbness, or a tingling sensation in hands or feet

There are several different types of surgeries that can be conducted for these conditions. The important thing to remember here is that these surgeries will be effective in removing the pain for a particular condition in an FM patient but will not be able to treat all symptoms of the disease. There was a time when FM was a medical condition that could only be treated through conventional medicines or drugs, but things are diverse today. Studies and research have been conducted in this genre to reveal several other procedures that are cost effective and highly reliable. The variety and flexibility of multiple alternative treatments for FM patients will also ensure they have more treatment ranges available that can help them to reclaim better health.[35]

Herbal Remedies. Insomnia, depression, and anxiety are interrelated, which means the existence of one problem can give rise to another or intensify the effects of another already present. For example, if a patient suffers from depression or anxiety there may also be sleep problems or disturbed sleeping patterns. There are several different types of OTC medications available for the handling of insomnia, depression, and anxiety. One of the most often recommended treatments is herbal medications. Herbal medications, often found over the counter, provide a safe and natural treatment for several FM clues including insomnia, depression, and anxiety. These remedies are available as teas, creams, supplements, and pills.[36]

Passionflower works very well for FM patients suffering from anxiety and insomnia. It can be consumed or applied in the form of liquid extract, tincture, tea, and infusion. Green tea is considered a top health drink worldwide and can provide relief from anxiety and depression. It also helps in increasing alertness and concentration while controlling blood pressure and stabilizing heart rate. Chamomile is consumed in the form of tea and provides relief from anxiety. St. John's wort is another herbal OTC remedy that is available in the form of pills, teas, and essential oils and is effective in the treatment of depression.[37]

Valerian is an herbal supplement that is highly effective for the management of insomnia in FM patients. Valerian is available in the form of sleeping pills and sedative medications such as benzodiazepines. Lemon balm is another herb for insomnia and also effectively reduces anxiety. California poppy is an efficacious herb for treating multiple FM symptoms, including mental and physical fatigue (neurasthenia), de-

pression, and nerve pain. It is also used as a sedative for people suffering from sleep-related quandaries. [38]

10

CONVENTIONAL TREATMENTS

Fibromyalgia (FM) is a chronic pain disorder with features such as debilitating and widespread pain. The causes are unknown, but the risk factors can be quite high, especially in women. It is known to coexist with other pain disorders such as rheumatoid arthritis as well as psychiatric disorders including depression and anxiety. Once FM has been confirmed, the first line of treatment governed by the family physician or internist is based on the nature and intensity of present symptoms. In the initial phases when the symptoms are not in a flared-up state, nonprescription or over the counter (OTC) medications can be quite effective.[1]

NONPRESCRIPTION MEDICATIONS AT A GLANCE

Most of the OTC drugs are used for procuring relief from muscle pain, anxiety, depression, and sleeping problems. The OTC medications vary according to the intensity of symptoms. Many of the common symptoms respond well to nonprescription medications.

Muscle pain and spasms are the most common symptoms in FM. This type of pain can be localized in nature or can be accompanied by widespread pain across the neck, shoulders, back, and legs. Fibromyalgia pain can vary from patient to patient and is usually described as a deep, throbbing pain or a dull, sharp ache. The pain is experienced mostly in the tendons, muscles, and ligaments in and around various joints. Most people suffering from this type of pain also experience a rise and fall in the intensity of the pain. The pain is either continuous or comes and goes, and it is often trailed by muscle cramps and spasms. Some of the most common OTC drugs for muscle pain and spasms include nonsteroidal anti-inflammatory drugs, acetaminophen, and topical pain relievers.[2]

Nonsteroidal anti-inflammatory drugs (NSAIDs), including ibuprofen and naproxen, provide relief from pain or aches caused by muscle stiffness. NSAIDs are also effective for reducing swelling, which is sometimes the primary cause of muscle pain. NSAIDs provide relief from pain by controlling the production of a hormone-like substance called prostaglandins, which are liable for causing pain.[3]

Acetaminophen, an effective OTC pain reliever, is classified as a nonopioid analgesic. Some of the commonly available drugs that contain acetaminophen include Tylenol, Anacin, Cepacol, Aspirin-Free Excedrin, Dristan, Ultracet, Zydone, Tramadol, and Oxycodone, among others. Acetaminophen helps to reduce pain by working on the sector of the brain that relays the messages related to pain. The recommended adult dosage of acetaminophen for patients suffering from FM pain is 650 mg every four hours or 1,000 mg every six hours.[4]

Topical pain relievers, available as analgesic creams, sprays, and rubs, can be bought over the counter. The topical pain relievers are dispensed on the skin to provide relief from muscle pain or ache, back pain, and joint pain. Different types of analgesics have different ingredients. The universally used ingredients in analgesics include capsaicin, salicylates, and counterirritants. Capsaicin is usually one of the primary ingredients and is apprehended to be the most effective. It is extracted from hot chile peppers and is most commonly found in skin creams. The application of capsaicin creams can cause a burning or tingling sensation, and it can take anywhere from a few days to weeks to find relief from pain. Salicylates is one of the main ingredients in aspirin and is also found in some analgesic creams. This ingredient is absorbed through the skin and helps in providing relief from pain in the knees, elbows, and fingers. Counterirritants cause a cooling or burning sensation when applied to the skin that helps distract the psyche from muscle pain. This category of ingredients contains several ingredients such as methyl salicylate, menthol, and camphor.[5]

SPECIFIC TREATMENT OF FM FATIGUE

Fatigue is another common symptom of FM, and it can be quite debilitating at times. Fatigue makes patients feel weak and exhausted, and a lack of quality sleep can extend the grogginess. There are three ways physicians can treat fatigue[6]:

- Medications, such as antidepressants, analgesics, and anti-inflammatory drugs can be prescribed.
- Exercise can have a profound and instant effect on insomnia, fatigue, and pain.
- Relaxation therapy, conducted by physicians or psychologists, is used to relax the mind and body so the patient can fall asleep.

SPECIFIC TREATMENT OF SLEEP DISORDERS IN FM

Sleep problems are fairly ubiquitous in FM and can range from difficulty in falling asleep to acute insomnia. The symptoms can also include frequent awakenings, in which the patient awakens disoriented. Some of the other sleep disorders experienced by FM patients include sleep apnea and restless leg syndrome. There are many patients who experience waking up feeling extremely fatigued, tired, or exhausted. They feel as if they have no energy. Normally, such people feel fatigued during the mornings and have an inclination to nap during the day. People suffering from FM also face a lot of difficulty concentrating. This type of condition is known as fibro fog. In such a scenario, physicians can help sort out the sleeping problems by following a treatment plan based on individual wishes. One of the significant aspects of FM is that the intensity and symptoms of the sleep disorder will vary from one patient to another. Also, physicians have to take into account the diagnosis of each patient while crafting a treatment plan that will suit the patient and will also be extremely effective.[7]

The management of sleep disorders in FM is done through medications and alternative therapies. Physicians often recommend sleep management plans that include medication and sleep modification[8]:

- Medications approved for the treatment of sleep disorders in FM include pregabalin (Lyrica), duloxetine (Cymbalta), and milnacipran (Savella). A range of other medications are also prescribed by physicians for FM patients that not only need help in managing sleep disorders but also other symptoms. These include muscle relaxants, pain relievers, and antidepressants.
- Sleeping habits and environment are the key factors of disturbed sleep often seen in FM patients. For example, a noisy environment can hamper deep sleep and break a consistent sleeping pattern. Similarly, erratic sleeping habits such as staying up late and waking up late can also be contributing factors. Physicians strongly recommend that patients change their sleeping habits gradually and try to extemporize an environment that will help them sleep better. Improving sleep habits and environment includes:

- creating an environment conducive to good sleep, including using a comfortable mattress
- a comfortable bed
- filtering the amount of noise and light that comes into the room
- maintaining proper room temperature
- establishing a bedtime routine
- avoiding caffeine prior to sleep
- using various methods of relaxation to induce sleep, such as listening to soothing music
- avoiding factors or things that create worry and stress
- exercising during the day (not close to bedtime) as it can make people feel energized
- limiting daytime sleeping as it will affect severely nighttime sleep

Patients suffering from FM can heal completely, though there is no absolute cure. In other words, experts have not found a way to make this disorder extinct from civilization. It is a situation that calls for a change in lifestyle and a proper treatment plan. It is important that individuals suffering from acute or chronic pain, lack of sleep, fatigue, and depression should inform their family practitioner or visit a physician to find vindication from FM symptoms. There are different treatment paths that can be followed singly or in combination to improve overall health and wellness.[9]

PRESCRIPTION MEDICATIONS

If OTC remedies are not enough to relieve FM symptoms, doctors can prescribe medications. The first line of action for most doctors is to prescribe an antidepressant, as these medications can help provide FM patients relief from pain, sleep problems, and fatigue. Apart from this, antidepressants play a prominent role in keeping depression at bay, which is a common symptom of FM. In some cases antiepileptics work well for the treatment of FM symptoms. For many years, tricyclic anti-depressants (TCAs) have been in use for FM treatment, particularly amitriptyline, which has become a pinnacle of FM treatment strategies. Of late, studies show that patients have developed poor tolerability to TCAs, and with advancements in research newer antidepressants are being stipulated for FM.[10]

Scientists in the last decade have conducted more than eighteen studies that involved more than 1,400 FM patients. Different classes of antidepressants were given to patients, and their recovery process was observed. Antidepressants prescribed included low doses of tetracyclic and tricyclic antidepressants, serotonin and noradrenaline reuptake in-hibitors (SNRI), selective serotonin reuptake inhibitors (SSRIs), and monoamine oxidase inhibitors (MAOIs). These prescription medica-tions are given to furnish relief from common FM symptoms such as sleeplessness, pain, depressed mood, and fatigue.[11]

These studies of FM patients revealed:

- The TCA amitriptyline (Endep and Elavil) was given to patients in low doses. TCAs had maximum effect on fatigue, pain, and sleep disturbances. After the administration of TCAs, patients were able to find relief from these symptoms.
- SSRI antidepressants (Paxil and Prozac) were administered to several patients with FM. These patients experienced a reduction in pain as well as a reduction in depression, although the medica-tion did not have any effect on insomnia or fatigue.
- SNRIs (Savella and Cymbalta) administered to patients did not provide much relief from depression, pain, or sleep disturbance.
- Monoamine oxidase inhibitors (Manerox, Pyrazidol, and Aurox) administered to patients provided a modest reduction in pain,

although there was no effect whatsoever on sleeplessness or fatigue.

Due to research findings like these, only specific drugs or medications have been approved for administration to patients suffering from FM. Individuals with FM are usually prescribed pain medication, muscle relaxants, antidepressants, and sleep-inducing goods. Over the years, the FDA has approved specific medications that can be prescribed by doctors to their patients to curb the various symptoms of FM. The various drugs for FM are classified as either SSRIs or SNRIs.[12]

Selective serotonin-reuptake inhibitors (SSRIs) are a division of medications that plays an important role in increasing the serotonin levels in the brain. A moderate rise in serotonin levels has several benefits for FM patients. The most common SSRIs prescribed by physicians for this disorder include Sertraline, Fluoxetine, Fluvoxamine, and Paroxetine. These medications also have a positive effect on other symptoms and help patients achieve improved sleep, reduce fatigue, and increase overall well-being. Physicians recommend SSRIs be taken in the morning. Some of the common side effects of SSRIs include nausea, agitation, and low sex drive.[13]

Serotonin-norepinephrine reuptake inhibitors (SNRIs) are more commonly known as dual inhibitors because they act upon two different chemical messengers in the brain—serotonin and norepinephrine. SNRIs are prescribed by doctors to FM patients to provide more consistent pain relief as compared to SSRIs. Some of the commonly prescribed SNRIs are Venlafaxine and Duloxetine. Studies have revealed that they are safe as well as effective for most patients, although they can have side effects such as vicissitudes in blood pressure and weakening of sexual function. These drugs are not prescribed to elderly patients as side effects can be serious. Some of the other side effects reported by patients include nausea and dizziness. Experiments reveal that Duloxetine has the ability to reduce FM pain by almost 30 percent. There are a few side effects of taking this medication, including dwindling appetite, dry mouth, nausea, constipation, increased sweating, sleepiness, and agitation.[14]

Another of the most common symptoms of FM is mild to severe fatigue. Severe fatigue can lead to chronic fatigue syndrome (CFS).

Fatigue in FM patients is sometimes related to lack of sleep and constant muscle pain or spasm. To oppose both fatigue and pain, doctors will often prescribe medication with multiple properties such as inducing sleep and pain reduction. Some of the most common prescription medications administered to FM patients apart from antidepressants include narcotics and anticonvulsants. Narcotics, for example Tramadol, are often imposed as they contain morphine or codeine. These medications not only provide relief from pain but also can help patients experience sound sleep. Anticonvulsants, also known as antiseizure medications, are prescribed to patients experiencing sleep issues and severe pain. It is extremely effective for dealing with nerve pain. The most commonly prescribed drugs in this category include Pregabalin and Gabapentin.[15]

Some of the other prescriptions drugs prescribed to patients suffering from insomnia include[16]:

- Suvorexant (Belsomra) is an orexin receptor antagonist. Orexins are a type of chemical that is involved in regulating the sleep-wake cycle. The chemical ensures individuals remain awake. Medications such as Suvorexant work by altering the action of chemicals in the brain, and this causes people to sleep instead of staying awake.
- Zolpidem (Ambien) is another prescription medicine that works effectively and helps FM patients get sound sleep. This drug works quite fast and can help patients to fall asleep within fifteen to thirty minutes of taking it. Doctors only prescribe Zolpidem to patients who are unable to get the minimum seven to eight hours of sleep. It is available in pills and an oral spray. The oral spray is called Zolpimist.
- Ramelteon (Rozerem) is a prescription sleep medication, which works in a different way than other sleep medications. It basically targets the sleep-wake cycle but does not depress the central nervous system while doing so. It is prescribed to FM patients facing difficulty in falling asleep. This drug is often prescribed to patients for long-term use.
- Eszopiclone (Lunesta) is another potent medication that is prescribed by physicians to FM patients suffering from insomnia. This drug helps people to quickly fall asleep. The drug can pro-

vide patients with sound sleep for the recommended seven to eight hours. The side effect of the medication is wooziness. The recommended starting dose of Eszopiclone is 1 mg per day.

- Doxepine (Silenor) is a sleep-inducing drug that is FDA approved. It is a prescription medication concocted for the treatment of insomnia in FM patients. It is also administered to patients who have disturbed sleep or wake up in their sleep. Doxepine helps people to sleep well by blocking the histamine receptors.

- Zaleplon (Sonata) is one of the contemporary approved sleep medications available to FM patients. The only drawback of Sonata is that it is active in the body for only a short period of time. This medication is not prescribed to persons who have a tendency to wake up during the night.

- Benzodiazepines are one of the most successful categories of prescription drugs used for the treatment of sleeping disorders encountered by FM patients. Some of the most commonly prescribed benzodiazepines include Restoril, Halcion, and Xanax. These drugs stay in the system for longer periods of time and can put people to sleep quite quickly. They are also prescribed as treatment of other sleep disorders including nightmares and sleepwalking. The biggest drawbacks of this category of drugs are the dependence it creates and the sleepiness that people report feeling throughout the day.

Doctors also prescribe different types of muscle relaxants to patients suffering from various muscle-related FM symptoms, including muscle spasms. Muscle relaxants help by reducing muscle tension and improving acute muscle pain, chronic low back pain, and increasing mobility. One of the most common muscle relaxants prescribed by doctors to accost muscle pain and spasm is diazepam (Valium), which helps by establishing relief from lower back pain that is commonly associated with muscle spasm. It is prescribed for short-term use due to the fact that it creates dependency. Recommended usage for this drug is limited to two weeks, and the maximum dosage is 5 to 10 mg once every six hours for severe back pain. Some of the other muscle relaxants that can be prescribed by doctors depending on the patient's needs and conditions include Soma, Skelaxin, Norgesic, Robaxin, and Flexeril.[17]

IMPORTANCE OF TAKING ALL SIDE EFFECTS OF BOTH OTC AND PRESCRIPTION DRUGS SERIOUSLY

Whether FM patients are self-administering over-the-counter medication or are using prescription medication, it is extremely important to know and understand the medications and the side effects they can produce. This gen is important especially when on antidepressants, as such medication can have severe side effects including sexual or erectile dysfunction and diarrhea or constipation. It is imperative that FM patients consider and properly understand the methodized side effects of all drugs prescribed for treatment. Every medication used for treatment of FM and most of its symptoms have side effects. The nature and degree of side effects vary not only according to the medication and dosage but also depend on the patient's overall health condition, tolerance level, and other drugs being taken. Some of the side effects can be temporary in nature and fade out with time, while others can be serious, including drug interactions and long-term side effects.[18]

A drug interaction is when two or more drugs (either OTC or prescription) react to another medication also being expended. Such a condition can arise when a patient is unaware of the interactions between their OTC and prescribed drugs. It is very important for the patient to inform the prescribing physician of any and all medications and treatments being taken. Drug interactions can be life threatening in many cases. Moreover, polypharmacy is a situation in which patients take multiple medications at the same time without discussing them with the prescribing physicians. Patients who compound their medication dosages without consulting the prescribing physician might be met with drug interactions. It is important to understand that drug interactions can have severe consequences. Drug interactions can not only have severe side effects but also can lead to death.[19]

Long-term side effects are another disincentive that FM patients might face if they do not take medication side effects seriously. It is the obligation of a doctor to inform patients about the side effects of medicines. For example, the side effects of antidepressants aimed at the treatment of FM, such as SNRIs and SSRIs, can include[20]:

- feeling sick
- experiencing an agitated state of mind

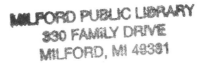
MILFORD PUBLIC LIBRARY
330 FAMILY DRIVE
MILFORD, MI 48381

- feeling anxious or shaky
- experiencing constipation or diarrhea
- suffering from stomach aches and indigestion
- suffering from repeated bouts of dizziness
- experiencing considerable loss of appetite
- headaches and migraine
- inability to sleep well or feeling sleepy throughout the day
- constant tiredness or fatigue

These side effects can be temporary in nature, but if not taken seriously they can also become permanent and can pave the road to other disorders. It is important for the patients to learn how to conquer the side effects. Only when patients know and understand the intensity and type of side effects they may experience when taking an FM medication can they trounce the side effects when they take hold. For example, if a specific medication produces side effects such as severe nausea and vomiting and if it continues for long periods, then OTC medications such as Benadryl can be used to provide relief from the side effects. Treatment of FM is possible in the modern age thanks to the range of treatment options available. Patients can opt to use over-the-counter drugs or can be given prescription medicines that will help them find relief from the pain and other symptoms embodied in the disorder. At the same time, it becomes extremely important to ensure that patients stay healthy and achieve overall wellness. This can be done not only through medication but also by developing a deep understanding of the medicines they are being prescribed. On occasion, something as simple as taking side effects of medicines seriously can be the single most defining factor between life and death.[21]

MORE ON CONVENTIONAL TREATMENTS BY PHYSICIANS

Once a patient has been diagnosed with FM by a physician, the next step will be to follow up with a proper treatment program. The physician plays an important role in engineering a program that will include different paths, including physical exercise, sleep strategies, various medications, and stress reduction therapy. At the same time, the physician also has to ensure that the patient is able to stay focused and committed to the program, as it will lead to overall improvement in FM symptoms and general health.[22]

Physicians will develop different treatment plans to treat individual patients according to the symptoms and severity of FM. There are several types of medications that physicians can prescribe to provide necessary relief from FM pain. The medications prescribed depend on the type of pain, location of the pain, and the intensity of the pain. The most common medications used include anticonvulsants, antidepressants, pain relievers, narcolepsy drugs, and sleeping aids. These medications are prescribed because they alter the patient's brain chemistry, and this helps in reducing pain, easing anxiety, providing relief from depression, and improving sleep.[23]

Physicians also recommend aerobic exercise along with medications to provide long-term relief from pain. Exercise is considered one of the most effective ways of treating FM. Exercise can provide relief from not only pain but also from sleeping disorders and fatigue. Aerobic exercises are highly effective in improving balance, maintaining bone mass, increasing strength, and easing stress. Physicians hold utility in creating an ideal exercise plan that can help patients control weight as a way to mitigate the pain caused by FM. The patient is advised to begin by walking five to ten minutes every day for a minimum of one week and to escalate the time by five minutes each week.[24]

11

FIBROMYALGIA AND DIET

A surefire pain relief diet has not yet been developed, but there are many things FM patients can do individually to find their own best diets. The interactions with medications must be considered when creating a diet that can alleviate FM symptoms. As with an exercise plan, patients should consult their doctors before significantly altering their diets. The patient must develop the habit of eating balanced, nutritious meals at regular times, and body hydration must be kept consistent to combat the symptoms of FM. If the patient suffers irritable bowel syndrome, a multienzyme tablet can help.

Change in an ever-adapting world has largely impacted the way we eat as well as live our daily lives, and this subsidizes the increasing rate of chronic diseases affecting all countries. Rendering an immense burden on the patient and family, chronic diseases are the main cause of deaths worldwide. Improvements in diet as well as the fitness of an individual can contribute in massive proportions to the decrease in such scenarios. Studies have indicated the treatment effectiveness of any medical condition is improved with the implementation of changes in lifestyle. The present-day "nutritional transition" from traditional plant-based diets to those that are elevated in animal fats and sugar, along with a sedentary lifestyle, are the underlying factors that influence the risk of the spread of such chronic diseases.[1]

Research has not yet determined a specific diet that would alleviate the conditions pertaining to FM. It is worth the patients' efforts to attempt to modify their own diets to improve the symptoms and the way they feel. From previous studies, tremendous information has been mustered in an attempt to figure out FM, the science behind this chronic disease, and its most effective treatment via diet. Doctors have been able to identify the role played by certain types of food that would support overall health.[2]

Intense sensitivity to a particular food, with this sensitivity varying from person to person, is a major cause of concern with FM patients. Some may be susceptible to dairy or eggs, while others cannot tolerate gluten and certain preservatives. Studies show that a small number of FM patients have symptoms worsen after eating certain foods. There are many more foods that fall under the hodgepodge of common allergens. Tracking food in a food journal along with reactions after consuming the food or food combinations is a good way to identify which foods aggravate specific symptoms. This helps patients clearly understand which ailments have negative impacts on well-being as well as those that had arrested symptoms of chronic pain and fatigue. This ensures a great deal of benefit to some patients from symptoms such as decreased pain and fatigue and an ease in irritable bowel syndrome symptoms such as constipation and bloating.[3]

Fibromyalgia is not a specific illness; rather, it is more of a gamut of symptoms that varies from person to person with different ailments presenting with a varying degree of severity. What may effectively work for one patient may not work well for another. If underlying conditions, separate from FM but also present, are treated, the FM client may find some relief from symptoms and feel an increase in overall well-being.[4]

An important factor that relates to diet is the mitochondrial dysfunction among FM patients. This dysfunction causes a lack of energy, which is a main symptom of FM. A diet rich in nutrients is important in order for the mitochondria to start begetting energy again. The higher the levels of dietary nutrients consumed the better the patient feels overall.[5]

People with FM benefit when significant nutritional changes are made. With the help of a nutritious diet and a healthy lifestyle, FM can be successfully opposed. There are a number of significant theories that help complement a healthy quality of life. These can be explored and introduced as therapies. Deep breathing exercises, yoga, or a good massage are generally effective and produce benefits. Not all patients with FM benefit from the same program. What works for one may not work for another. Each one experiences inimitable symptoms or combinations of symptoms that contribute to this being a difficult condition to diagnose and treat. It is essential that each patient tailor dietary changes to their personal experiences.[6]

FOOD AND DIET PATTERNS

Of the many different diet plans, determining what food categories to avoid and what to include on a regular basis is the most effective way to prevent FM symptoms. The chronic pain and fatigue symptoms will eventually reduce when this plan is executed consistently. This tried and tested method will work exclusively for the individual who eliminated foods successfully. Unlike standard medication, this diet has to be solely determined and heeded by the patient to significantly see improvements in symptoms as well as overall health. Studies of many diets in relation to FM concluded that elimination diets worked best to promote a stress-free condition with fewer symptoms. The FM patient has many new diet plans to choose from, such as the Paleo diet, South Beach, and the Ayurvedic diet. The Paleo diet uses mostly uncooked and raw food and could trigger irritable bowel syndrome in some people. In the South Beach diet, the cooking process breaks down food to an elementary form and extinguishes the parasites, microbes, and fungus, thereby ensuring they do not infiltrate the body. The patient's liver and detoxification system is free of overload, and there is no excessive demand on the body for the zinc and magnesium that the organs use while detoxifying.[7]

Patients with carbohydrate intolerance or reactive hypoglycemia (low blood sugar) that occurs after eating carbs have to be cautious about the excess insulin that is absorbed into the muscles and liver and stored as fatty acids in the cells. Protein diets are suggested as they decrease cravings, help shed weight, control hypoglycemia, and increase energy levels and reduce feelings of lethargy. An ideal diet consists of 30 percent carbohydrates, 30 percent fat, and 40 percent protein, though as professed the conditions and nutrient needs vary from person to person. The popular Zone diet works well because of the reduced calorie intake. The idea of a low carb and high protein and high fat diet works effectively, especially with moderate functional fitness.[8]

People who have fibromyalgia should choose a diet with plenty of protein while reducing carbohydrates to regulate the body's blood glucose level to a stabilized state. The fluctuation in the blood glucose levels elicits fatigue. A "heart healthy" diet, low in saturated fat and high in fresh fruits and vegetables, contributes to a healthy core. This type of diet plan contributes to overall health, giving the body better capacity to cope with any disease. Studies have shown a significant response to a vegetarian diet composed of raw whole foods leading to a reduction in FM symptoms. The Mediterranean diet eliminates sugars, which in turn avoids sugar rushes and reduces fatigue. A low glycemic diet helps dislodge symptoms and restores the energy that helps the patient think clearer. This diet is good for both the physical and mental agility of the person with FM.[9]

FOODS THAT CATER TO FIBROMYALGIA

Several types of food promote the well-being of those with FM, while others can worsen the condition. Small decisions to make healthy lifestyle choices could improve the patient's total well-being. Choices such as eating small, frequent meals through the day can drastically elevate energy levels, as well as snacking on protein. Breakfast should by all means include some protein and whole grains. Boiled eggs and oatmeal are a good start to the day and will prevent blood sugar from spiking and give quantum energy to kick-start the day in spite of bodily aches and feeling lethargic.[10]

Omega-3 fatty acids are found in foods such as fish oil, walnuts, and flax seeds. Eggs are also sources of healthy fat and have been shown to have an impact on inflammation. Cold water fish and walnuts have anti-inflammatory properties, and though they may not offer relief from pain they contribute to a healthy heart and are most definitely a worthy addition to any diet. Eating oily fish or linseeds for their anti-inflammatory properties is a good dietary addition.[11]

Fruits and vegetables help combat oxidation stress pertaining to inflammation. Good choices are colorful foods such as grapes, beets, and carrots. A diet packed with fruits and vegetables outfits the body with additional nutrients and antioxidants. Nutrients such as calcium are found in deep green vegetables, and malic acid is found in apples.

These antioxidants are beneficial for reducing the destructive effects that cause tissue damage, which is the effect on the tissues when the body generates reactive chemicals called free radicals. An excess of these free radicals leads to tissue damage and contributes to vivid pain and increased fatigue levels.[12]

Nutritional and vitamin supplements, in addition to a healthy diet and a reasonable fitness level, have benefitted people with FM. Melatonin, for instance, has been known to significantly improve the quality of sleep, while vinpocetine, an extract from the periwinkle plant, has been shown to improve brain functions. Supplements such as these help support muscle function and reduce fatigue and gastrointestinal distress.[13]

The body needs an abundance of magnesium. Adding refried beans to the diet will provide extra magnesium. Fresh foods, preferably organic and free from additives, preservatives, and commercial dyes, should be introduced.[14]

CONTRAINDICATED FOODS

People suffering from poor sleep often consume too much coffee, leading to an oversensitive bowel. In some cases, wheat-based food when consumed frequently also account for bowel sensitivity. In addition, FM patients should avoid tea and nicotine as they are stimulants and antinutrients.[15]

MSG added to some foods is a known cause of insomnia. Excitotoxins such as aspartame affect the nervous system and are known to stimulate the pain receptors and cause increased pain and sleeplessness. Aspartame, commonly used to make sweetening agents such as Equal or NutraSweet, causes more physiological glitches and magnifies the symptoms of FM.[16]

Mental fog and fatigue are caused by dehydration. Drinking sufficient water helps reduce headaches and backaches significantly. This is a common factor that is generally overlooked.[17]

Patients are advised to eliminate or at least reduce salt and sugar as well as stimulants and antinutrients. Excess salt intake can cause tight muscles and calcium retention to occur. Sugar is known to cause bloating and fatigue and lowers immunity. Cutting out simple carbs, sugar, and fructose may not cause an impact on FM, though it could significantly reduce the risk of yeast infection that may be causing secondary pain. Fungi thrive in products such as white bread and cakes that can contribute to the pain. Cutting out high fructose corn syrup and sugar in particular can make a difference in such patients.[18]

Another major noticeable change is seen when carbonated drinks and beverages sweetened with fructose are eliminated. The carbonation causes a metabolic reaction that results in the sugar entering the blood more quickly. This sudden rise in blood sugar followed by a subsequent drop leads to an energy deprived, fatigued condition. A drop in energy level creates more craving for sugar, and then again, a drop in energy and fatigue. Studies have suggested that the sugar in carbonated beverages may contribute to yeast problems. Carbonated beverages are said to leak phosphorus from the bones, and the aspartame in sodas introduce memory loss. This cycle in no way helps to reduce fatigue and related pain. Owing to the drop in energy levels, caffeine-rich beverages are often sought after as a source of energy. The boost in the energy received is false, and the brief high energy will subsequently fall to a substantially lower, deprived, deep sedative state. This sedative effect makes the resulting tiredness all the more powerful. Cutting out caffeine can significantly improve energy levels, and the difference is almost immediate.[19]

Common allergens such as eggs, dairy, wheat, and citrus can occasion a decrease in health quality. Cutting out yeast and gluten yields two enunciated benefits. The two ingredients generally appear inextricably in baked goods, so cutting one typically cuts the second. The overgrowth of this yeast fungus in the body can cause muscle and joint pain in people with FM. Gluten intolerance, a condition created by the excess of gluten and the inability to break down the protein, results in digestive problems and other stomach ailments. Fatigue is also associated with gluten intolerance.[20]

Avoiding dairy products may lower the symptoms associated with FM. On the other hand, if milk does not cause negative symptoms, drinking a skimmed version is a fat-free alternative that will build salubrious bones from the calcium and lean muscle from the protein.[21]

The more than two hundred species of plants listed as nightshade plants, such as bell peppers, eggplant, tomatoes, and chile peppers, are known to trigger arthritis pain (due to solanine). If these vegetables do not trigger FM pain, patients should not restrict these from their diet as they are very nutritious.[22]

DIET-RELATED RESEARCH AND FIBROMYALGIA

There is very little in the form of research findings on nutrition and diet for FM patients, so little is known about the food categories that is best or which should be avoided. It is known, however, that a well-balanced diet nurtures good health and healing. A low-fat diet with high-immunity-boosting antioxidants will work simultaneously to maximize the alertness and energy levels with minimum fatigue and muscle pain. Making the necessary modifications to lifestyle and diet are sure ways to eliminate its symptoms. Adding exercise and stretches, good exposure to the sun, and plenty of water (a minimum of eight glasses a day) to a nutritious diet plan will help overcome fatigue and pain.[23]

Caffeine in soda and other beverages acts as a diuretic and requires that the patient drink additional water. Research has shown that caffeine accounts for the loss of calcium through the urine at a faster rate than if none were consumed. This also consigns immense stress on the adrenal glands and on the liver. Due to chronic stress and inadequate nutrition, FM sufferers may have adrenal malfunction. The adrenal gland releases a surfeit of adrenalin that leads to acute symptoms and is responsible for panic attacks. Therefore, caffeine and carbonated drinks should be avoided.[24]

Avoiding fried and salty foods helps reduce pain and swelling among FM patients. This includes bottled juices and sodas that use preservatives, salts, sugar, colorings, and additives. Chocolate should be consumed in moderation as it is high in fat and caffeine.[25]

At the more scientific level, through the body's natural processes, cells receive nourishment while eliminating waste. It is normal to crave processed foods, sugar, starch, and fat when transitioning to a healthy lifestyle. This is common among all people, not just those with FM. Taking extra care to eat well-balanced meals is essential to those with this chronic disease. Eliminating one food type at a time and by making gradual changes in lifestyle can make the transition easier. Eating well in moderation and by incorporating an overall change in eating habits with variety and balance reduces fatigue and maximizes energy levels.

Introducing fresh vegetables and fruits to the diet creates a shielding effect on any chronic disease, including cancer and heart diseases. The phytochemicals present in fresh produce have a protective effect and help combat diseases. These phytochemicals reduce the response to pain among FM sufferers, providing required relief. Incorporating raw or partially cooked fruits and vegetables into the diet improves the quality of life for anyone, with or without FM. Avoiding foods that aggravate the FM condition thereby eliminates the symptoms and contributes to a better quality of life.[26]

Thus, the symptoms reported by FM patients, including long-term chronic pain, inflammation, swelling, memory problems, stiffness, difficulty in understanding concepts and conceptualizing, and the mental characteristics of moodiness and emotional woes, are all preventable with this healthy approach. The benefits of a healthy diet to either cater to the people with chronic diseases such as FM or to impart a healthy lifestyle depends exclusively on the addition of certain food categories and the elimination of others. The rationale behind a health diary is to discern and identify personal triggers of FM symptoms while concurrently learning the foods that ease symptoms. Overall, patients can improve their quality of life and ensure a healthy existence by upholding a healthy diet.[27]

12

IMPORTANCE OF EXERCISE IN THE TREATMENT OF FM

It has been generally thought that brain activity spearheads the bodily response. Those diagnosed with nervous system disorders often feel depressed, tired, and physically distressed, and the first logical solution would be to rest. However, recent research has proven otherwise. New studies claim that the brain and the body have a reciprocal relationship, which leads researchers to conclude that exercise can significantly benefit mental health in FM.[1]

The brain is the most complex organ known to mankind. It learns, grows, and changes with the functions of its environment. Experts conducted an experiment that involved the correlation between aerobic exercise and the functions of the nervous system. The results showed a positive interaction between physical activity and the hippocampus, the part of the brain that is responsible for learning and storing memories. There was a significant effect on the long-term memory of subjects in comparison to the control group. The scientists believe that exercise can lead to better creativity and imagination.[2]

Once folks reach their late twenties, brain function tends to decline, which leads to memory loss, emotional instability, and other neurological and psychological dysfunctions. Since mental activity is something that cannot be controlled, it is essential to focus on what can be altered. Exercise is essential to mental health for several reasons. Just as what people eat can significantly affect their thoughts, activity can produce an equivalent response. New research shows that physical exercise is just as important as mental exercise. When a person moves, certain functions of the brain are turned on, and the process of learning actually begins. As a result, the mind functions efficiently, giving the body the proper signals to act on throughout the day. Positive brain development also involves the bodily release of a plethora of hormones, which is necessary for the aid and production of brain cells. In contrast, according to a study by researchers at the Wayne State University School of Medicine, inactivity can become detrimental to mental health and may cause more problems than what patients are already experiencing.[3]

A study from Stockholm also concluded that the production of new cells in the hippocampus has actually helped the brain develop antidepressant effects. Exercising causes the muscles to produce a protein called PGC-1 alpha that breaks down the substance kynurenine, which is primarily a result of stress.[4]

With these new findings, people with neurological disorders must now give a considerable amount of thought to physical activity. However, other factors should also be considered to exploit the benefits of exercise since some neurological illnesses can increase pain if applied with limited research and a lack of medical guidance. Patients who continually experience muscular pain often think it's best to avoid exercise at all costs. As it has now been shown that pain is a neurological reaction, inactivity can actually aggravate the situation. Adding proper low-impact aerobic exercises to daily activities can be helpful in dealing with symptoms and ripening the brain's understanding of pain.[5]

THE BEST EXERCISES FOR FIBROMYALGIA PATIENTS

Physical fitness has been a strong go-to option for people seeking relief from FM. The goal of trainers is to introduce an active lifestyle, to reduce the pain and other responses, while being aware of certain limitations and allowing their clients to accept the limits of their condition. Research has proven that a sedentary lifestyle only contributes to worsening symptoms, showing that lack of exercise is equivalent to overexertion, especially when it comes to overcoming the confines of pain.[6]

However, exercise is not a direct treatment for FM. It only helps prevent symptoms from worsening. That is why patients must strive to maintain a consistent physical routine rather than focusing on short-term goals that often result in overexertion and disappointment. So before committing to any kind of bodily exercise, patients must set expectations for something that is achievable in due time.[7]

Walking. Walking is a light aerobic exercise that increases blood circulation, improves overall stamina, boosts energy levels, and reduces pain and stiffness. In addition to these bodily advantages, walking also has beneficial effects on the brain. Walking reduces stress and mental decline. When suffering from mental disorders, stress can be one of the major triggers that can worsen the symptoms of the illness. Patients are advised to avoid as much stress as possible. Walking can increase the body's production of norepinephrine, which moderates the body's response to stress. Moderate walks can also increase memory and delay mental decline. A study by researchers from the University of California revealed that women sixty-five and older who walked regularly have better memory retention than those who walked less often. Walking improves sleep, and people who move more suffer less insomnia. Five to six hours of movement a day will increase body warmth. When the temperature returns to normal, it signals the body to become sleepy. Walking also alleviates depression by releasing endorphins naturally produced by the body. Endorphins are a linchpin of happiness and euphoria. In fact, thirty minutes of walking boosts the moods of depressed patients faster than antidepressants.[8]

Yoga. Yoga exercises concoct mind and body balance. Yoga focuses on relaxation and stress reduction. In a new research study in Oregon, it was revealed that women age twenty-one or older showed significantly greater improvement in FM upon participating in yoga exercises. It aids the body's coping mechanism against pain, and also lead to a better mood in patients and keeps them calmer and less likely to succumb to hormonal changes. Yoga boosts memory, helps concentration, and blocks out the noise of the environment, allowing the patients to clear their heads and reflect on just a single thought. Staying calm allows the mind to function at its optimum pace. Yoga also mitigates the effects of post-traumatic stress disorder (PTSD). Women who have gone through physical abuse or a serious amount of pain that has left a considerable mark on their personalities commonly experience nightmares and flashbacks. Hatha yoga has been proven to be a therapeutic antidote for patients suffering from PTSD.[9]

Aquatic Exercise. When discussing traditional forms of healing, soaking in warm water is considered one of the longstanding types of treatments. Warm water therapy has engendered significant improvements in patients suffering from musculoskeletal diseases, which include FM. Exercising in a warm pool can help improve breathing and loosen joints, resulting in prolonged relief from pain. Warm water also downgrades inflammation and swelling and has also been proven to improve emotional health and sleep patterns. Warm water helps drive down the pain caused by chronic diseases such as FM. Swimming, especially in warm water, can promote the movement of affected areas without aggravating symptoms. Aquatic exercises have had more health benefits for patients experiencing chronic pain than any other type of physical exercise. A study conducted by researchers revealed that women who did exercises in warm water for eight months experienced a commodious improvement in the major symptoms of FM. This includes pain, stiffness, anxiety, depression, and other factors. [10]

Biking. The circular motion of bicycling can contribute to good blood circulation, and being in the fresh outdoors can certainly uplift any mood. However, one thought that FM patients and caregivers must consider when biking is their choice of equipment. Patients should find a bike with a stable seat and a sturdy frame to avoid falls. This low-impact exercise is also beneficial for cardiovascular health. Biking is a weighty "antidepressant." As the wind blows through their hair and the wheels rush forward, cyclists tend to enjoy a sense of peace and relaxation. This sense of peace and improved relaxation is due to the production of endorphins and cannabinoids (the same chemical that is released when marijuana smokers are under the influence), which improves mood. It is said that as a person pedals his or her bike, more nerve cells are forced to fire. As these neurons light up, they produce compounds, such as *noggin*, that allow the synthesis of new brain cells. This doubles the usual production of new cells. Biking also allows the release of neurotransmitters, which are the messengers inside the brain. These allow the new brain cells to communicate with the old ones for a fast and efficiently functioning nervous system. Biking also creates a "younger" brain. Neuroscientists report that people who exercised for three months had the brain volume of those three years younger. This significantly contributes to overall well-being. Not only is exercise beneficial for those suffering from FM and other chronic diseases, it is now a noteworthy step for those trying to overcome it. [11]

Pilates. Pilates can help in the rehabilitation of FM in a number of ways, including improved muscle strength and stability, created through a discipline of relaxation and control. However, one of pilates's major advantages in dealing with FM syndrome is its promotion of breathing and breath work. When patients practice breathing exercises, the blood's oxygenation results in an increase in circulation in all areas of the body, which helps deflect tension away from the muscles. The production of brain-derived neurotrophic factor, which most scientists commonly refer to as the "Miracle Gro" of the brain, is buttressed through the practice of pilates. This allows a patient to be smarter and take more control of the mind. Just like any other form of relaxation exercise, pilates promotes good sleep. It relieves the brain from stressful thoughts and helps produce positive emotions that not only prevent insomnia but also leads to lengthier and more comfortable sleep periods. Pilates causes deeper muscle activation. The body and brain work in sync. Another fact patients should keep in mind is that every time they move, specific areas of the brain produce certain functions. Pilates and its deep-core activation promotes the use of involuntary muscles in the parasympathetic nervous system that individuals may not be even aware exists, sending signals to areas of the brain that haven't been used. The result is a fitter nervous system and a possible hike in pain threshold. [12]

THE WORST EXERCISES FOR FIBROMYALGIA PATIENTS

Patients experiencing FM symptoms should use care when choosing a new exercise routine. Excessive exercises that strain the muscles can increase pain rather than reduce it. Some activities to avoid include running and jumping, extreme neck exercises, hiking, dancing, aggressive strength training, and overexercising. [13]

Running and Jumping. Fast, sudden movements can stir up pain associated with FM. These swift actions strain the muscles and possibly cause swelling in the joints. Although some people have been able to continue with these activities, it is better to take the extra precaution and consult a doctor if planning to exercise by sprinting or jumping. Of course, incorporating these exercises are not entirely impossible. To determine if workouts are being overdone, patients can test whether or not it is possible to carry on a conversation while running or jumping. Caregivers should remember that FM patients use exercise for the sake of relaxation and not solely for the sake of sweating out toxins.[14]

Extreme Neck Exercises. The neck is probably one of the most critical tension areas in the body. Even just sleeping in the wrong position can cause an average person an enormous amount of discomfort from neck pain. Neck pain can lead to chronic headaches and trouble sleeping. Exercising the neck is advisable, but only with proper precautions so as to not aggravate the problem. Therapists also do not suggest neck massages as this area is very vulnerable and could greatly damage the nervous system's connection to the spinal cord. Head banging is one neck activity that a patient suffering from FM should avoid. The sudden and swift action of the head can unfortunately engender intense dizziness and muscle strains.[15]

Hiking. While walking produces great results, lengthy hikes with a heavy backpack is an extreme activity and is usually not advisable for people who suffer chronic pain. Although the great outdoors is good for relaxation, putting too much weight on joints could likewise cause more pain. Fibromyalgia patients should mainly avoid walking in the mountains. If patients do decide to saunter in mountainous regions, it would be wise to bring a walking stick or something similar to help keep the tension off the knees and other sensitive joints.[16]

Dancing. Although it is true that there are professional dancers who have FM, continuing with this type of exercise might not be entirely beneficial. Aside from belly dancing, which has been proven to help ease pain, other forms of dancing can involve terse movements and stiffness in some areas of the body. Dancers, who use the art to express themselves, usually do not exert control and neglect the limitations of their bodies. This can lead to an increase in physical fatigue.[17]

Aggressive Strength Training. Studies have been published that have actually recommended weightlifting as one of the best exercises to combat FM. So why is it in the list of worst exercises? Light strength training can be beneficial, but it is easy to overdo it. With so many possibilities of worsening symptoms instead of alleviating them, experts say that this is one of the exercises that must be avoided when first incorporating workouts into daily routines. If patients are determined to add hard-line strength training, they are advised to work out a safe plan with their physical therapist. They should begin with two to three pounds for no more than ten minutes a day and no more than three times a week. Once the patient is ready for more, they should lengthen the time of the workout. Increasing the weight load can definitely be detrimental to an FM condition, especially if not done within the guidance of experts. Again, the goal is always to keep a balanced mind and body.[18]

Overexercising. Exercise is good, but too much exercise can be adverse for FM patients. With insufficient precautionary measures, overexertion can lead to increased pain and reduced mobility. Improper posture can also aggravate FM symptoms. The best plan of action is to start at a unhurried pace and gradually accrete the activity level. Patients should also be aware of their body's limitations in order to avoid any negative reactions. People often ask the question of how much is too much. According to professionals, the best way to identify what works for each individual patient is to choose one specific exercise routine and stick to it. It might be wise to get the advice of fitness luminaries before entering any program that claims to be auspicious for FM sufferers. They can definitely advise patients as to which particular activities are best in targeting individual pressure points. Patients often experience different amounts of pain in various regions of the body, so physical therapy should be intended to suit those needs.[19]

When dealing with chronic pain diseases, one should never forget to strike a balance between the body and the mind. Breaking down workouts to shorter periods of ten minutes each will help enhance mental and physical health rather than engaging in heavier physical activities. Beginners should begin with three to five minutes of gentle activity and gradually work up to more physical activities. Exercise for the purpose of losing weight is different from exercise with the goal of paring down pain. This is not a competition, and there is no calendar or weight scale to determine whether or not a patient has had any progress. Again, it all boils down to relaxation and self-satisfaction. Patients with FM can get the most out of exercising by being patient and gathering enough information. Fibromyalgia patients all have different body types and different pain responses, so it is necessary to plonk limits based on individual needs. If in doubt, patients and caregivers should seek the advice of a physical therapist.[20]

13

LENDING A HELPING HAND

Every day is an endeavor to overcome a multitude of obstacles. Youngsters need to devote time to school and studying well enough to earn passing grades. They also feel stressed from peer pressure because of wanting to belong in a group, not to mention the overwhelming stress they might get from the worst kind of dilemma one could possibly experience in school: bullying. As for adults, life just becomes even more complicated. All the problems in school seem to be multiplied as an adult. There is the struggle of a typical work life, which includes not only physical but also emotional stress. Being an adult and trying to maintain a balanced life can at times simply seem to be quite a challenge. With just one additional plight, life becomes even more challenging. That is what happens for people with debilitating FM. Like any other problem, patients feel better when they know that they are not alone, that another person also knows and cognizes how they actually feel.[1]

That is why, as unfortunate as it may sound, knowing someone who is also diagnosed with FM can help to alleviate the emotional pain a patient is going through from this disease. No other person can relate better to an FM sufferer than another patient. A fellow sufferer knows how it truly feels to wake up every morning wishing all of these symptoms were just a nightmare or that finally this abysmal disease would simply disappear and life could be less challenging again. Only a fellow sufferer knows how hurtful and annoying it actually is when a person without FM, who may not know the patient very well, makes a comment about FM or gives unsolicited advice on how to treat the symptoms—advice that the patient probably already knows anyway or, even worse, something that is completely unfounded. Oftentimes only a fellow sufferer knows what it is like to go through the daily motions of life masquerading and convincing themselves that everything is okay, that everything is as it should be.[2]

With or without FM, it is all a matter of having a positive outlook because, after all, life will be what the patient makes it. The reality is sometimes that the incapacitating effects of FM can be overwhelming. There are just days when there is such unbearable physical pain that the patient simply wants to give up. Teens may not want to go to school anymore, not only to avoid dealing with the stress of maintaining good grades but also to sidestep having to explain what they are going through to peers. These peers might not accept the explanation anyway or, worse, they might just ridicule FM and the student runs the risk of becoming the target of bullying. An adult, having to work to sustain a living while having a bout of excruciating pain from FM is something a patient does not even want to think about. These are just a few of the undesirable situations that make it difficult to always keep a positive attitude. Some days, FM sufferers just want to mope and concede defeat simply because that is how they truly feel, and only an equal can completely understand that.[3]

IMPORTANCE OF SUPPORT GROUPS

Finding comfort with kind-hearted people in a support group is one helpful way to conquer this often challenging disease. However, even if others who are not afflicted with this disease do not actually know how it feels to be diagnosed with it, it cannot be denied that they, too, can be of great help. As long as there are people who are caring and kind enough to empathize with the patient, they can be of real help to the patient in not having to go through this battle on their own. By getting involved in a support group for patients diagnosed with FM, a person can express all of his or her emotions, thoughts, and concerns without having to fear if others in the group will cast judgment. Instead, the main concern is to simply be there for each other, to listen and to offer a positive environment to give friends and themselves a break from daily challenges. In these support groups, members can vent about any worry, no matter how big or trivial it may seem. Through them, a patient's disconcerting thoughts will have a place where they will be silenced because in these groups there is always assistance to help deal with any problems or concerns a member might be having.[4]

The simplest, but definitely not inferior in value, form of assistance the group can give is listening. This action may not seem like much to others, but for those going through difficulties, having people who will listen to you without judgment can definitely alleviate the sadness because instead of having to carry all that weight of sadness alone, with the presence of a support group there will be people who will help carry the burden. Through the help of support groups, patients can also bid farewell to the feeling of being unaccompanied because these people will simply be there for each other to make everyone feel that they belong in a family suffused with compassionate and good-hearted people who accept each other for all that they are. Fibromyalgia patients may not be perfect, may not be able to do some of the tasks that most others can do effortlessly, but they do not need to worry because these support group members understand. No one will magnify shortcomings or offer criticism. They will simply be together. After all, they are called a support group for a very good reason. They offer their company to guarantee to each patient that they are there to help in whatever way they can, to the greatest extent that they can. They may not endure the same collection of symptoms, but they assure each other that they will fight this battle unceasingly together.[5]

Fibromyalgia in itself is already stressful, but for most sufferers, another cause of stress is the mounting financial burden that it poses. As is scientifically established, FM is a chronic disease, and that means that the battle is lifelong, until of course a cure is finally retrieved. Until then, afflicted patients need to live with the truth that FM is going to be costly in terms of care and management. So this is where support groups also offer their help. They will do their very best effort to provide the financial assistance needed to make this disease more manageable. They will try to connect you with the right doctors who can help you manage this disease by providing a suitable treatment plan, including the right medications and therapies.[6]

Yes, being afflicted with FM is like living in a bad dream, but even though this is the case it is still not the end of the world. Those stricken with this condition must always focus on the positive. That is why support groups also celebrate all the members' triumphs, joyful moments, and accomplished goals. To them, there is no little or trivial success story. Every success is worth celebrating. Just the fact that everyone got to live one more day to be with family and loved ones is a success in itself. These support groups will help patients shift their focus from the negative to the positive. As much as it is possible, they will help create a more optimistic outlook despite the cloud of negativity that FM can bring now and again. With an improved outlook, the patient will be able to appreciate all life has to offer. Living with FM is not easy and it is most definitely not a pleasant experience, but despite this, support groups will still help because they do not want anyone to give up on the FM battle. In times when almost everyone connects through the Internet, it is not at all difficult to find a support group for people with FM. For someone who is not able to physically attend a group meeting, there is the preference of online support groups and message boards. Having this option to talk with other FM patients online is also helpful for people who have busy schedules. Through online support clusters, the patient does not need to leave the comfort of home to keep connected with other people also going through this illness. There are advantages and disadvantages to both online groups and local community groups, but as long as patients make the effort to enlist a support group, they are already helping themselves win the fray against FM.[7]

HOW CORPORATIONS CAN HELP

Health insurance providers or disability insurance companies can really help FM patients by changing how they categorize FM from a mere disorder to an actual disease. Since there remains controversy within the medical community regarding the cause and nature of FM, insurance companies are likewise skeptical about FM and view it as only a minor disorder. As a result, many patients or sufferers of this illness are denied long-term disability benefits. In addition to the physically debilitating effects of the illness itself, this kind of denial of health benefits is a blow to afflicted sufferers. Fibromyalgia patients, especially those with severe cases, are facing tremendous challenges sustaining a professional occupation. The pain they experience due to doing physical work in their jobs makes it almost impossible for them to retain long-term commitment even if they desire to. In addition to their pain hindering them from sustaining a living, they are finding it difficult to afford long-term medical expenses for medications and therapies to steer them away from their disease.[8]

This denial of fair health benefits by many disability insurance companies has been an ancillary complaint among people suffering from this disease. Fibromyalgia sufferers and insurance companies have not been seeing eye to eye when it comes to what the right health benefits are for those afflicted with the disease. On the insurance companies' part, the extent of the benefits they will provide to the patient will depend on the patient's disability test results, such as the Functional Capacity Evaluation (FCE). There is a major flaw with this particular kind of disability test because data is only collected during the test period. As such, the test fails to acknowledge the reality that FM patients also experience pain and other symptoms for several hours after the actual physical exertion concludes. This delayed onset of symptoms or flare up is a real problem many patients go through. Therefore, it would be just and unquestionably logical for disability insurance companies to start considering the fact that the FCE is not enough to provide a strong guideline for the extent of the health benefits they are willing to grant. It is high time they keep in mind that FM sufferers also experience delayed flare ups. To settle this discrepancy, it is fairly reasonable for insurance companies to include subsequent information after the actual testing of a patient's disability. Thus, after a patient is subjected to the FCE, information regarding his or her response and functioning should still be gathered and recorded. This inclusion of subsequent information creates a clearer picture as to how sapping this disorder actually is.[9]

HOW THE GOVERNMENT CAN HELP

Eventually, the government is the one entity than can create the biggest impact in the match against FM. The government is created for the people. So when the people, in this case those afflicted with FM, are in need of help, who better to rely on than the government? One form of abetment that the government can provide is, of course, more financial aid. Since FM is a long-term illness, patients suffering from it are fraught with the dilemma of a lifetime of medical bills. This is where a more justified allotment of people's taxes should come in the picture. A portion can be allotted to provide FM patients with the means to brook a more manageable life in spite of the setbacks they are dealt from having this illness. They should be aided in being connected with the suitable medical experts and having access to the right kinds of therapies, such as physical therapy or cognitive therapy. They should also be provided with the right medications needed to manage this disease. It might be impossible to provide a lifetime supply of free medications for every FM patient, but at the very least, the government could find a way to make these medications more affordable for them. After all, these patients often find it knotty to work long term due to their weak endurance when it comes to physical work, and they also cannot mentally function as well as healthy people because their concentration is affected by the pain accompanying this disease. Earning and sustaining a living is difficult for FM patients, and that difficulty is compounded even more when adding expenses from the long-term use of medications.[10]

Moreover, the government could be of help to FM sufferers by creating more readily accessible support groups, perhaps by making sure that there is a FM support group in locations where people could easily get to it. These support groups must also be effective in providing assistance to afflicted patients. Thus, the counselors must not only be knowledgeable of the disease but they should also be compassionate enough to empathize with what the patients are going through. The government should also strive to encourage afflicted patients; this could be done by fashioning advertisements for various FM support groups.[11]

Another effort from the government that would be helpful to afflicted patients is spreading information and awareness concerning the disease. Right now, not everyone knows exactly what FM is. Some may not have even heard of it at all. Thus, it is important that the government educate the public about this very real disease. The actual causes of it may still be uncertain, but it is important that people, especially those vexed by the disease, receive the right information about it, such as what triggers it, what exacerbates it, and how to manage it. The government could also found public advisories to have the information more readily available to the public.[12]

Finally, what would make a tremendous impact in the wrangle against FM is continuously funding research programs on this disease to shed more light as to what really causes it. There is more data than ever before about this chronic illness. If research endures, study centers will uncover more crucial information about FM, and maybe soon they will be able to discover a cure. As long as the government continues to fund these types of research studies, there is anticipation for a one-stop solution to FM. The battle against FM may be long, but it is a fight that should not be impractically surrendered. People suffering from this disease do deserve to find the light at the end of the tunnel. They deserve to regain the life they once had before stumbling upon this disease. In essence, once a cure is found, all the other intricacies associated with FM will be forever abolished.[13]

IV

Iron Will to Face Fibromyalgia

14

APPROACHING THE MENTAL ASPECTS

There exists a myriad of approaches by which an FM patient can better cope with stints of depression, self-pity, and anxiety. First and foremost, a patient must consult with a health professional or a mental health specialist for a psychological evaluation. Once diagnosed, there are several methods of treating depression, which include psychotherapy, medication, and self-help techniques.[1]

Also known as talk therapy, psychotherapy helps FM patients manage pain and deal with illness by transmuting their outlook or perception about situations. The two main types of psychotherapy that are thought to be most effective in treating depression are cognitive-behavioral therapy (CBT) and interpersonal therapy (IPT). Counseling is another favorable option.[2]

Also known as mental health counseling, CBT can be very effective in suppressing mental disorders and in managing the stress and anxiety of FM patients. In this method, a mental health counselor speaks with a patient following structured and systematic procedures. This can help patients identify negative thoughts and dysfunctional emotions and address inaccurate feelings and maladaptive behaviors, thereby aiding patients to handle and respond to challenging situations more appropriately. Cognitive functions help FM patients change their way of thinking about pain and enable them to fare through pain more effectively. Normally, a CBT program requires regular face-to-face sessions with a therapist for a certain period. Cognitive behavioral therapy may be effective for mild to moderate depression. On the other hand, it may not be the best option for some, particularly those with severe depression.[3]

The IPT approach is a short-term action that aims to address interpersonal issues, focusing on symptoms related to the patient's personal relationships, particularly with loved ones, family, and friends. Interpersonal therapy does not focus on resolving personality issues but on relationship issues, with an emphasis on identifying problems specifically involving a patient's interaction with others.[4]

Another popular type of psychological therapy is counseling. This may be conducted in group sessions or one-on-one talks with a therapist. In counseling, a patient is encouraged to share his experiences and thoughts. During these sessions, patients may find some subterfuges to better cope with pain or handle other issues related to FM symptoms. Although group therapy has many benefits, individual therapy is regarded as a more effective process.[5]

Antidepressants mainly affect the brain chemicals serotonin and norepinephrine—the neurotransmitters responsible for regulating and enhancing mood. On the other hand, while antidepressants are generally effective, they may have adverse side effects, so the prescribing physician should closely monitor a patient taking antidepressants. Selective serotonin reuptake inhibitors (SSRIs) are among the newest and most commonly prescribed antidepressants for patients suffering from FM and are generally regarded to have fewer side effects than other types of depressants. Most popular SSRI drugs include fluoxetine, paroxetine, citalopram, and sertraline chloride.[6]

Serotonin and norepinephrine reuptake inhibitors (SNRIs), another type of antidepressant, function like SSRIs by easing out depression symptoms, such as irritability, erratic temper, and sadness. These are also ordered for the treatment for nervousness and nerve pains. Among the SNRIs ratified by the Food and Drug Administration are duloxetine, venlafaxine, and desvenlafaxine. Patients who are in a severe stage of FM are primarily treated with tricyclic antidepressants (TCAs), which work by altering the brain chemicals to alleviate depression symptoms. Some TCAs include amitriptyline, amoxapine, doxepin, trimipramine, and protriptyline, which are available in liquid form. Side effects have been observed in some FM patients taking TCAs. These include dry mouth, vision problems, and exigency when urinating and moving bowels, drowsiness, and profuse sweating. Other adverse effects include erratic heartbeat, tremor, and decreased sex drive. Because of the severity of these side effects, TCAs should be meted with care.[7]

Since some FM patients feel that they can manage other FM-related symptoms more effectively if their physical pain is more bearable, pain-focused FM treatment may then be very beneficial. In this approach, tramadol and acetaminophen are commonly prescribed to provide relief. However, these should be taken with caution and only under the supervision of a doctor.[8]

Getting sufficient sleep and rest is vital when treating FM. Due to pain brought about by FM, a patient may have a hard time sleeping or may have fragmented sleep, thereby tampering with the natural body clock or the circadian rhythm. Studies show that sleep deprivation has negative effects on mood. Good sleep habits are crucial for a person with FM. Therefore, getting enough rest, having a regular sleep routine, and systematizing daily activities can be beneficial in eliminating depression associated with FM.[9]

People who suffer from mild to moderate depression may gain from meditation by clearing the mind of negative thoughts and elating their positive mood. Playing soft and soothing music may also be helpful. Engaging in some relaxation and mind-calming techniques, such as tai chi or yoga, is proven to be beneficial for some patients. Being in the company of loved ones and people who can be a source of inspiration and encouragement is a good way to beat depression. Furthermore, an FM patient should maintain an open communication with family and trusted friends and openly share feelings with a confidante. Engaging in physical activities, such as low-impact cardiovascular exercises including walking, jogging, and riding a bike, can be very beneficial.[10]

Exercise not only has physical benefits but mental benefits as well. Getting enough sunshine and natural light is a great mood lifter. A sufficient amount of bright light will help boost mood and may help regulate sleep patterns. Getting a walk outdoors, basking under the sun, breathing fresh air, or just simply enjoying nature can be very beneficial for beating depression and for bolstering overall mental and psychological health. Reading inspirational books or watching movies with an upbeat story line can be uplifting. Watching comical or inspirational films will help boost the frame of mind and encourage positive thoughts. Following a healthy, balanced diet plays a crucial role in treating depression and other FM-related symptoms. Starchy and sugary foods should be avoided; instead, a patient should eat more green and leafy vegetables and fruits such as pineapple and banana, which are considered to be serotonin-enhancing foods. Too much caffeine tends to squelch the body's production of serotonin; therefore, drinking coffee should be minimized, if not avoided. It is strongly advised that FM patients eat three full meals a day and avoid skipping meals. Depression is curable, however, but immediate treatment is important. Thus, the deceptive trappings and symptoms of depression must be identified at the early stage, through proper knowledge and education about this condition.[11]

APPROACHING FIBROMYALGIA-RELATED MOOD SWINGS

Fibromyalgia contributes to biochemical imbalances in the brain, the primary cause of mood swings. There are three main approaches for addressing erratic moods or mood swings related to FM—lifestyle modification, alternative medicines, and medications.[12]

Modifying lifestyle and habits is the foremost approach to addressing mood swings. This entails self-discipline, but this method is the most cost-effective and has the least risks. Simple changes in lifestyle can alleviate mood swings and promote overall physical health. Diet plays a vital role in managing one's mood since food affects blood sugar levels. For example, consuming too much refined sugar and drinking coffee may temporarily fortify a person's mood, but the feeling will then drastically drop when the sugar high wears off. Similarly, alcohol may make someone feel better in the short term but may result in further mood problems later. Therefore, it is imperative to have a healthy, balanced diet and to achieve and maintain an ideal body weight. Complex carbohydrates, such as wheat, bran, and oats, can bump serotonin levels. Likewise, protein-rich products, such as meat, fish, poultry, and dairy, may better an FM patient's mood. Studies show that eating magnesium-rich foods also has a connection with mood as well as with energy levels and muscle pains. Thus, it is also advisable to have sufficient doses of magnesium in the daily diet. Drink water to keep the body hydrated. The recommended amount of water intake is at least eight glasses per day. Instead of drinking sugar-laced energy drinks, drinking a lot of water is the best option. Water flushes out toxins from the body, keeping the digestive system healthy. [13]

A good night's sleep is an important factor in managing mood swings. While a person suffering from FM may have difficulty sleeping due to pain, it is beneficial to establish a regular sleep routine. Developing a calming and relaxing routine before bedtime, such as listening to soft music, reading, or taking a warm bath, may contribute to good sleep. Also, making the room conducive for sleeping by keeping it dark, cool, and free from any distractions can make a difference in achieving a sound sleep. It is important to have a minimum of seven hours of sleep each night and maintain a specific time for sleeping and waking. Since caffeine is known to be a stimulant, it is recommended to drink no more than one cup each day, or drink decaffeinated coffee instead. Alcohol can also interfere with sleep; therefore, it is recommended that the patient refrain from drinking alcohol close to bedtime and limit red wine to one glass per day. [14]

Regular exercise is essential in mood management since it stimulates the release of endorphins, known as the "happy chemicals," in our body. Physical fitness is vital in successfully managing FM. An ideal fitness program for FM patients is composed of stretching and low-impact aerobic exercises. Stretching should be done regularly and at least a few minutes once a day. Ideal aerobic exercises include walking, bicycling, and swimming, which truncate the possibility of severely straining the joints. While exercise is essential for FM patients, it must be done properly. Simultaneously constricting and extending muscles or an eccentric contraction will lead to muscle soreness. Therefore, activities such as blow drying hair, vacuuming, gardening, walking down stairs, among others, must be discouraged. [15]

Spending time with loved ones, family, and friends has many positive effects on mood. Time spent with loved ones tends to boost levels of oxytocin, also known as the "love hormone," which acts as a brain neurotransmitter. Listening to radiant or inspirational music plays an important role in mood management. Studies show that music helps raise people's mood. Soothing and soft music tends to relax the nervous system. [16]

Alternative methods are usually safe and can be very effective in managing erratic moods. There are several options, such as herbal supplements, massage, and acupuncture. There are two main types of herbal supplements—phytoestrogenic, which are beneficial in addressing estrogen deficiency; and hormone regulating, which promote the body's hormone production. Phytoestrogenic supplements can counteract a lack of estrogen and thereby address mood swings. However, prolonged use of these supplements may burke the body's natural hormone production, which could result in a drastic decline in hormone levels. Hormone-regulating supplements appear to be the best option for many as these are effective and have the least side effects. On the other hand, there are some supplements that have not undergone research as thoroughly as prescription medications for safety and efficacy. It is therefore very crucial to consult with a doctor first before taking any supplements because there are some that can have adverse effects if ingested with other drugs.[17]

One of the most well-known herbal remedies for addressing mood swings is the Hypericum perforatum or St. John's wort, which affects the brain's neurotransmitters. However, St. John's wort can have severe interactions with other prescription medicines, so it is best to consult with a doctor prior to using it as a therapy. Prescription drugs can be very effective, but they also involve the highest risk. It is therefore advisable that FM patients consider the option with the lowest risk, such as lifestyle changes, before traversing to the next level of treatment or medication.[18]

APPROACHING FIBROMYALGIA-RELATED ATTENTION LAPSES

The importance of adequate rest and sufficient sleep cannot be overemphasized. Sleep deficiency is attributed to short-term memory, irritability, and inability to focus. Fibromyalgia patients should preserve a stable circadian rhythm and have regular sleeping patterns to promote a healthy sleep hygiene. Fibromyalgia patients are advised to refrain from eating too much processed foods and instead eat a balanced diet consisting of complex carbohydrates and protein and generous servings of fruits and vegetables.[19]

Keeping a note pad handy to jot things down to help remember important information and record thoughts and ideas can be very effective. Making a to-do list to keep track of motions to be done is very helpful. Mapping out and listing the things to do and setting priorities are crucial so as not to divert attention to other less important things. Since the human brain can only handle two tasks simultaneously, adding another one can result in a poor output. Therefore, FM patients should avoid multitasking and instead focus on one task at a time. Fibromyalgia patients are advised to work in a quiet environment that is free from distraction. However, if a patient cannot work well in a very quiet setting, playing soft music in the background may be helpful. Some studies also reveal that classical music may aid in sharpening focus. Loud music, chatter, and unpleasant sounds and noises must be avoided as these tend to disrupt cognitive functions. Further, several studies have linked watching too much television to depression and a regression in mental alertness and overall physical health. Therefore, TV time should be kept to a minimum. Fibromyalgia patients should strive to perpetuate focus and avoid things that may divert attention from the task at hand. Taking short breaks in between tasks is good for FM patients, particularly if engaged in time-consuming tasks. Stretching, taking a stroll, getting something to drink, and breathing fresh air outside can be beneficial in improving mental alertness. Nature tends to calm the senses. Studies reveal that breathing fresh air, basking in the sun, or just simply appreciating the beauty of nature can have a significant effect on memory, attention, and focus. Accomplishing tasks need not be a sole undertaking of the FM patient. Delegating some responsibilities to other competent, trusted individuals may be helpful.[20]

APPROACHING FIBROMYALGIA-RELATED MEMORY LAPSES

Since cognitive problems are attributed to tiredness and overactivity, FM patients are advised to refrain from strenuous or mentally draining activities. Taking frequent ten-to-fifteen minute breaks is also encouraged to boost mental alertness. A well-rested body and mind can increase productivity. Therefore, FM patients are advised to get enough sleep and avoid sleep deprivation. It is advisable to have a regular sleep routine to maintain circadian rhythm. Since FM patients may have difficulty sleeping, sleeptime rituals are recommended, such as taking a warm bath before bedtime; keeping the bedroom cool, quiet, and conducive for sleep; drinking a warm glass of milk; and listening to soothing music. Some FM patients who also suffer from *restless leg syndrome* may have difficulty sleeping. In this case, the doctor might prescribe *dopamine* agonists to ease out anxiety and pain. Power naps, or short naps, particularly if a person is able to dream during naptime, can help recharge the brain, boost mental alertness, and enhance overall cognitive ability.[21]

Since the brain needs nutrients to perform efficiently, proper nourishment is a must. Some foods, such as whole grains, leafy green vegetables, oily fish, and nuts, among others, can actually enhance memory and brain functions. Omega-3 fatty acids can be very effective mind boosters. There are also spices that are known to improve memory and enhance cognition, such as cinnamon, sage, cumin, and cilantro. Foods rich in omega-3 fatty acids include salmon and tuna, walnuts, and flaxseed oil. Multivitamins and mineral supplements may also be opportune for FM patients. The micronutrient choline can help further a patient's mental performance as well. Choline-rich foods include eggs, legumes, dairy products, chicken liver, and fish. Proper hydration keeps the brain functioning well. Not only does drinking water keep the body hydrated, but it is also good for the skin, maintains a healthy digestive system, regulates body function, and promotes general physical health.[22]

The importance of regular exercise and physical activities cannot be overemphasized. Exercise promulgates oxygen to the brain, thereby enhancing concentration and memory. Walking, aerobics, and dancing are some of the most beneficial forms of exercise that can enhance the cognitive functions. Studies reveal that exercise enhances the hippocampus, the brain component involved in cognition and memory. The recommended length of exercise is about thirty minutes each day. Fibromyalgia patients are advised to consult with their doctor prior to engaging in a new workout. Listening to music while working out can also improve memory.[23]

Stress has negative effects on the cognitive faculties of an FM patient. A person who is stressed out will find it difficult to think or recall well. Likewise, extreme negative and positive emotions may cause cognitive concerns. For instance, a feeling of happiness may activate the production of *adrenaline*, which can have an adverse effect on cognition. Therefore, it is necessary to avoid getting stressed, properly control emotions, and abrogate the adrenaline rush to be able to think clearly. Avoiding negative thoughts and emotions, maintaining a positive attitude, and being optimistic despite ordeals could be one of the best approaches to managing memory lapses. A good laugh can do so much for the heart, for the brain, and for the entire body. Laughing arouses the brain and overall cognition.[24]

Studies claim that listening to classical music can improve memory and boost cognitive functioning. Likewise, listening to informative podcasts can help stimulate the brain. Most FM patients experience memory lapses when they are overloaded with multiple tasks. Multitasking may be counterproductive. Finishing one assignment or task at a time will be more effective. Since people have different levels of alertness at different times of the day, it is important that an FM patient choose the best time of day to perform most efficiently. Most FM patients feel that their brains are at their sharpest during the morning. The key therefore is to choose the most appropriate time of the day to perform important tasks that require memory and concentration.[25]

Relaxing and calming activities, such as yoga and tai chi, can help improve memory, dispose of stress and anxiety, and promote better sleep. Reading plays a paramount role in cognitive function. Reading nonfiction, inspirational, or self-help books not only sharpens the memory and improves cognition but also motivates, inspires, and heightens knowledge. Talking to others, particularly about relevant topics, can improve cognitive skills. Socializing can also have a positive impact on memory and cognition.[26]

A more organized home or workspace can enhance productivity. It is difficult to think well in a disorganized, chaotic environment. Minimizing clutter, arranging things in order, and putting things in their proper place may help avoid undue stress and panic and enhance memory and cognition.

There are medications adjudged by clinical research scientists for treating memory lapses and cognitive problems. There are also some alternative medicines that claim to boost mental alertness. However, there are medications that may have adverse effects in the long run; thus, they should be taken with care and under the supervision of a doctor. Some medications for FM patients can actually affect cognition and memory; thus, it is best to consult with the doctor to recommend medicines with fewer side effects.[27]

Fibromyalgia is a clinical condition that can have a colossal impact on the patient's quality of life. However, through proper and sufficient understanding of this condition, along with the right and proper approaches, FM can be managed. Managing FM is an everyday undertaking, which may initially seem insurmountable. Nonetheless, proper management and treatment, amalgamated with the patient's sinewy self-discipline and determination, can make this condition more bearable and could eventually result in better health.[28]

15

BEING A PARENT WITH FIBROMYALGIA

Parenting is one of the most challenging parts of life. It is the stage of life at which a person must put the needs of family and children above all else. It is a time of crucial decision making in order to be able to provide the necessities while also having a productive life. Being a parent is also an enjoyable part of life. Yes, parenting is a gift, but some parents face challenges. This is especially true when the parent, whether the mother or the father, suffers from a chronic condition such as fibromyalgia, a disease that affects the central nervous system.

WHY BEING A PARENT WITH A CHRONIC CONDITION CAN BE DIFFICULT

Fibromyalgia is challenging for parents. Some parents are able to cope, but others fail to see the brighter side. This is because they are filled with the exhausting "work" of being a parent. They may have done what needs to be done for the day, such as doing the laundry, cleaning the house, and other chores common for parents, but because of their disease, they need to rework their plans. The most difficult problem FM patients face is accepting that they have the disease. Why did it choose me? The wife or the husband with the disease will undergo denial, anger, bargaining, depression, and acceptance, but it is important for all patients to remember they did not choose the disease, nor did it choose them. It is normal to go through these different stages of grief, and it is important for the patient's partner to understand each stage. It is helpful for both partners to go to the doctor together so that they can both understand the diagnosis, symptoms, and treatments. The patient may ask themselves, "Why me?" This is often traced by a list of things that could be accomplished if only there wasn't this diagnosis. As the partner of the affected parent, it is important to understand the feelings and moods an FM patient is likely to go through. Be present, listen, and provide support.[1]

Two of the stages, anger and denial, sometimes occur simultaneously. The patient will be angry with just about everything; it might be about the simple things that can no longer be done or the executions of directions; for example, the errand of cleaning the dining area to be done by the eldest child. The FM parent might be enraged because he thought the child performed the task but it was not done appropriately. Then the next day, the FM parent will try to prevent more anger by doing everything rather than delegating tasks. Fibromyalgia parents will continue to do errands and chores, pretending that they don't have the disease. Other family members may try to stop the FM parent from doing everything, but they push them away, saying, "I can do this, I am not sick." Deep inside, there is anger because the FM parent no longer feels effective.[2]

"Can the ground just swallow me up?" As a parent it is very important to be able to fulfill the needs of the children. Having a chronic disease can prevent the parent from doing so, leading to depression. This is the most difficult stage of grieving. The FM parent feels helpless and cannot fulfill parental duties. Family members can offer to console the FM parent, offer help and guidance, but the FM parent often wants to push them away. If these feelings of helplessness and depression are not dealt with effectively, they can lead to thoughts of suicide and scarpering away from the family. If the patient is able to cope, then that can result in a more positive acceptance of the disease, and therapy and medications will be more likely to be effective. Why is FM so difficult? A chronic illness has incalculable effects on the ability to parent effectively as well as to carry on the proceedings of daily life. The FM parent can experience difficulty performing normal, everyday tasks. They might notice a transformation in actions and behaviors toward themselves and their families. They may compare themselves with their partners or other parents, and look back at activities they were previously able to do. They may try to do things they want, but the pain is limit-ing.[3]

LIFESTYLE DIFFERENCES BETWEEN A HEALTHY PARENT AND A PARENT WITH FIBROMYALGIA

It is difficult for others to notice or identify a FM parent from a healthy parent. A person with FM looks no different than a person without it. Although everyone appears the same, the parent with FM can indeed see the difference. There are certainly a lot of variations between a healthy parent and a parent with a chronic condition.[4]

The Healthy Parent. All parents have skills to nurture their child. They can communicate with their child as often as needed, with the thought of the welfare of the child always a foremost concern. They can set and follow the structure or rules that they decide on as a couple to build their family and to give their children direction in life. They can perform their normal daily routines for their children. They can use the available resources in their environment to make their family healthy, most especially for the healthy parent (someone who doesn't have a chronic condition). They don't need to worry about themselves first before their family.[5]

A healthy father can provide financial stability to his family. He is able to work and do errands at home. He can play with his children, as well as caress his wife. Supporting his family is his main priority; maintaining his health and his family is part of his daily affairs, and having time with his friends and time for himself to do his hobbies are part of his growth. Problems may arise, but he can solve them alone or togeth-er with his wife and family. He can get sick; however, these conditions are usually just the common ones that can be easily cured. Overall, his lifestyle is something that is customary for the community.[6]

A healthy mother is one who can take care of her family. If she is a working mom, she needs to find balance between her work and main-taining the home, especially for her children. If she is a stay-at-home mother, then she has ample time to make her home the best place for her family. As part of her lifestyle, she can plan and prepare the meals, do house chores with ease, and have time for herself. She is at peace because she can care for her family, and provide them with all their needs. For example, she can fix their breakfast and pack lunch boxes for her school-aged children, clean their uniforms or school clothes, and maintain the cleanliness of the house. She can even look good doing all her chores and hobbies. Being a mother might be a busy task, but she is very good at multitasking. This is the lifestyle that she gladly embraces as a mother.[7]

The Ill Parent. Added to the challenges and duties of being a parent is having a condition that is unbearable when not properly understood and accepted or properly treated or managed. Fibromyalgia parents worry about not being able to provide for the necessary needs of their family and may be afraid of losing their family. Once diagnosed with a chronic disease such FM or another chronic pain or chronic neurological disease, there will assuredly be lifestyle changes.

If the father is the one with the chronic disease, he needs to adjust his work to fit his condition. At first it can be a very difficult transition; he might need to stop working for a while. Once he is able to cope with his sickness, he can resume working. However, there will be changes like taking his medicines on time. He also needs to change his physical activities to minimize the occurrence of pain. He is able to play with his kids, but some activities may be limited. The FM father also needs to take time for himself. It means that he needs to give himself "me" time. This will help him to relax his body and mind. Of course, regular check-ups are needed in order to routinely assess his condition. The household chores will never be the same again, if the mother is the one having the chronic condition. She might tarry in bed more often rather than doing chores around the house. She might be awake early in the morning to prepare the family's breakfast, but it is not at the usual pace she used before the onset of the symptoms of the disease. She needs to be able to cope with her condition, accept it, and understand it. The family should also understand the condition, so that help in doing the errands at home can be divided among the other family members. She should not exhaust herself; instead, she should learn relaxation techniques. Allowing time for herself and undergoing treatment should be balanced.[8]

OTHER CHANGES IN LIFESTYLE

Fibromyalgia parents have more decision making to do than healthy parents. They need to be careful of their actions as they can affect their condition; they have to make conscious choices every day. The daily schedule should be carefully thought out to make sure that even the simplest details will not be forgotten. This kind of planning is to make sure that everything the FM parent does in any given day will not cause a breakdown, discomfort, or a flareup of symptoms. A chronic disease can be so unpredictable that a patient might have a very good day followed by a really bad day. If the FM parent begins to feel a flareup or reprobate times coming on, the daily schedule may have to be adjusted to make the day easier. For example, if the FM patient needs to prepare dinner for the family but is experiencing a flareup of symptoms, another option will have to be considered. A choice might be to order food from a delivery service or ask the healthy parent to pick up takeout. Keeping a health journal or diary can be helpful. The patient lists symptoms or triggers, along with anything that helped provide relief.[9]

Doing so will allow the patient to track what did or did not work. It is also important not to dwell on these bad days; instead, the FM parent must keep a positive outlook and remember to focus on the good things that also happen. Having a sense of gratitude in small areas can help keep moods elevated. Using sticky notes around the house or office can remind the FM parent to keep a positive attitude. For example, a note on the kitchen refrigerator of a smiley face could remind the FM parent and other family members to smile. A note at the front door that says, "Have a good day," is another example. Another deflection that should be made is in relation to expectations. This one can be difficult to accomplish, since FM patients might be tempted to think in terms of "what if," or "I wish," or "if only." It is normal for FM patients, whether or not they are parents, to compare themselves to others if they have not yet accepted their diagnosis. It is a good idea to join support groups; they will help with tips on how to change a viewpoint or perspective. Lastly, changes may need to be made with regard to handling the children, especially if they are infants or toddlers. When looking after the children, it may be easier if they are limited to certain areas. This will make it easier to watch the children and sit for a rest if needed. Fibromyalgia parents will need support so that family exigencies can be solved and the needs of the FM parents can be met. [10]

HOW TO RAISE CHILDREN AS A FIBROMYALGIA PATIENT

One important thing to remember is that different stages in the children's growing years means that there will also be different needs and adjustments for the FM parent. Raising a child starts from pregnancy, but being a parent does not stop once the child reaches adulthood. The discomfort felt by mothers who have FM may be exacerbated by pregnancy, but with proper medications, FM should not prevent a couple from constructing a family. [11]

Infants. Crying is the primary form of communication for the infant; they convey a lot of meaning in different types of cries, such as being hungry or expressing discomfort. The parent will be able to recognize the different sounds of crying that their child makes for each need. The needs of the infant can disrupt the normal routines of the parent. This is veritable even in pregnancy; for example, the unborn child can impact the mother's sleep cycle. In cases in which one of the parents has a chronic disease such as FM, the spouse needs to be aware of the responsibilities of caring for an infant in order to offer support and help. For example, if the mother is unwell, then the father needs to be aware of how to change diapers and feed the infant, and he should be the one to wake up during the night to provide care. [12]

Toddlers. The biggest challenge with toddlers is that they are very active. They want to try to learn new things either with the help of a parent or by themselves. During this stage, the parents usually show the toddlers how things are done, and they learn mostly by mimicking the parent. Toddlers want to be independent and can become frustrated if their expectations are not met. They begin having tantrums at this stage from frustration. A judicious approach is now needed so that the FM parent's bad day from the chronic disease will not clash with the tantrums of the child. The parent with FM should be careful of the behavior he is brandishing onto the child. He should prevent this clash between them, for example, by letting the spouse or another adult relative watch over the children. Also, since the toddler is learning, it is good to teach him about the condition, especially for ages three and up, who can understand simple elucidations. In this way, the child will also be careful with his actions toward the parent having the disease. [13]

School-Age Child. This is the stage at which the child wants to prove that he can help and be responsible at home or in school. They can build friendships and play independently. They learn both at home and in school. Since there are new environmental factors that affect the behavior of the child, proper parental guidance is really needed. The child is now ready to accept responsibilities at home, and can appreciate explanations about your disease. As a parent having the condition, it is important to balance being a parent and a parent-teacher for a child. Being a guardian, one must let the child help with the house chores and explain their importance, and why the help was warranted. This will encourage them to help the family, especially you. If you are a stay-at-home mom, it is good to let them experience how to prepare their lunch boxes and how to fix things. Be careful not to be anxious if they have done something differently from your expectation, or did not do it correctly. Remember that stress can trigger your disease. It is better that your spouse help you in teaching your child to do the chores, so that when you are no longer feeling well, then you can just relax for a while. If you are the father, the challenge is how you will be able to discipline your child. Anger should not be your resort when your child is performing differently. You can talk to your spouse about ways of disciplining and setting rules in your house; it is still your job to be the decision maker of the family, but it does not mean that you should be the implementer as well, because it might trigger your pain. A parent-teacher role is mainly to edify the child after school, helping them with their homework and projects. The psychological symptoms of the disease may lead to the inability to help them with their schoolwork, unless the parent is already undergoing therapy and medications that will tail off the discomfort. So it is recommended that the healthy spouse be the one to assist the child. [14]

Adolescents. The teenager needs a lot of guidance and supervision in order to prevent them from doing things they might regret. They are on the path to look for their own identity and their place in society, but they are still being held back and seen as a child by some people or their own parent, which can lead to role confusion. They form groups or peers that influence their actions and behaviors. They want to be free and to experiment with their bodies. They also receive a lot of pressure from what their parents expect and what their "world" expects. To be able to raise adolescents properly, all family members should set directives, as well as the consequences for disobeying the rules. Everyone should understand these rules, especially the adolescent. This will also lessen the burden the parents will feel if their child does something inappropriate. Gratitude should also be noticeable. Since there will always be bad days when an individual has a chronic disease, unpretentious acts of goodness should always be praised so that the bad day will turn out to be a good one. If the FM patient occasionally lets the child make decisions on his own, as long as he knows the values, the child will acknowledge the responsibilities he needs to come to terms with.[15]

16

FIBROMYALGIA-RELATED OCCUPATIONAL CONSTRAINTS

Fibromyalgia can greatly affect professional and private life because it affects social interaction. Some individuals who suffer from full-blown FM while in the midst of their careers have ultimately stopped working as a result of hurdles with performing normal tasks. However, it is not impossible to lead a professional life regardless of uncertainties and the obstructions brought about by this disorder. Currently there is no known cure for FM, but there are medications available that doctors can prescribe to help manage the symptoms. There are also methods a patient can use to prevent or subjugate the onset of the symptoms, thereby managing it so as not to disrupt their daily activities, including their work.[1]

SPECIFIC WORK-RELATED ISSUES CAUSED BY FIBROMYALGIA

Is it possible to still be able to work even with this disorder? Yes. In fact, many doctors believe that patients suffering from FM should not treat this disorder as a disability. Studies have also shown that patients who have ceased working have the tendency to also stop doing regular activities during the day and therefore get less exercise. They are also likely to lose contact with friends or coworkers and eventually forgo a sense of purpose in their lives. This can cause patients to feel more depressed and frustrated, and these negative emotions can only make other FM symptoms even worse. There are many FM patients who continue to work either on a full-time basis or at part-time jobs. Fibromyalgia is not a progressive illness, and it is not a life-threatening condition. Physical activities will not cause harm to those who suffer from FM; in fact, it can be deemed helpful in some cases. However, it cannot be denied that recurring physical pain, fatigue, or brusque symptoms will make work a challenge for those with the disorder. Some challenges that patients may experience while trying to lead a professional life despite the presence of FM can include memory problems and concentration loss; reduced productivity; sensitivity to the work area; and anger, anxiety, and depression.[2]

MEMORY PROBLEMS AND LOSS OF CONCENTRATION

Many patients experience fibro fog at some point in their illness. Those who find themselves under a fibro fog often experience forgetfulness and a lack of focus. They will tend to become perplexed and will struggle to seek mental clarity. One of the causes of fibro fog, or brain fog, is a lack of sleep, which is also something brought about by FM. Insufficient sleep tends to dilute memory, judgment, and attention. Fibromyalgia patients who are working professionals find it particularly frustrating when they have trouble remembering when the next meeting is, figuring out what they need to do next, and focusing to complete a job assignment. They can sometimes become indecisive and cannot be expected to make sound judgments during a stressful or hectic discussion. Some patients report having trouble coming up with the correct words to use and at times will end up stuttering or tend to say one thing but actually mean another. Most patients find that having fibro fog greatly limits their mental ability to attend to regular job tasks. Because patients generally have trouble sleeping, fibro fog is one trigger for depression. Doctors can prescribe medications to help patients deal with insomnia and depression. Unfortunately, most of these medications contribute to brain fog. Patients who are experiencing fibro fog are advised to avoid operating heavy machinery or driving to prevent accidents.[3]

REDUCED PRODUCTIVITY

Even just getting up every day can prove to be a real struggle for FM patients. The pain felt by each patient may vary in intensity. It is by personal evaluation of pain levels that patients are able to determine whether or not they are capable of going about their normal workday. The onset of pain for FM patients is unpredictable. Some patients find it tormenting to perform normal daily work activities such as writing, reaching out to pick up a piece of paper, or even just sitting. Patients who experience joint pains as a result of FM may have trouble doing actions such as walking short distances, bending, lifting objects, lightly pushing or pulling, and other work-related activities that require any degree of physical exertion. This greatly impacts work speed, productivity, and the ability to deliver completed projects on time.[4]

There will be times when there will be increased workload, and therefore the job will become more demanding than it usually is. Some employers or coworkers may also show less consideration toward workmates suffering from FM. This creates a rise in stress level and working pressure and may trigger some of the symptoms of the disorder. Pain is perhaps the worst symptom of FM. It is what most often keeps a patient from being productive. Stress is a huge trigger of the pain symptom. For some patients, getting that job promotion equals a higher level of stress, and a higher level of stress equals frequent or possibly heightened inceptions of pain. Because of this, some patients become less and less motivated to work or to further their callings because of the thought that it will prove to be either too difficult or impossible.[5]

SENSITIVITY TO THE WORK AREA

As it is a given that most of the symptoms of FM may affect a patient's ability to perform physical work at times, it is also important to note that patients may also suffer from sensitivities to light, sound, temperature, and even to certain odors. These elements can bring about pain. People who suffer pain sometimes have an automatic cognitive response as to how they will cope with it. More often than not, patients tend to avoid any situation or environment that they perceive to be something that would either trigger or aggravate their symptoms. Almost automatically, like stimuli, the patient wants to have less to do with the situation that is most likely to cause them more pain. Having a tough discussion with the boss, getting held up in a long meeting, or when the boss demands too much and employees end up overworking themselves are common scenarios that ensue in most workplaces. For those who suffer from FM, these situations may seem like one more challenge to have to deal with, and they will tend to shy away from it out of fear. What kind of fear? There's fear of triggering symptoms, fear of not being able to do well, and fear of being criticized or called out for their imperfections. If this emotional fear is left uncontrolled, patients may tend to feel threatened by their friends and by their workmates. They may retreat from most social or work-related activities. This will create an even bigger distance between them and their psychosocial environment. Such situations will often lead to depression due to isolation and low self-worth.[6]

ANGER, ANXIETY, AND DEPRESSION

More often than not, people who suffer chronic pain are also suffering from depression. The inability to perform properly at work is quite frustrating for most patients who are leading a professional life. The impact of their disease on their work affects their own professional identity. Inaptitude for normal tasks as well as someone in a lower or equal position reduces the patient's self-esteem, and there is a constant fear that arises with the thought of losing the job that they value. It is unsurprising that before and after being diagnosed with FM, patients often use an increased amount of sick leave. The constant pain may sometimes be debilitating and affect daily routine. In particular, jobs that require a lot of physical work will be a difficult challenge. Having supportive employers and coworkers who are willing to accommodate changes and fine-tune the work assigned to be less stressful but still be productive can boost self-esteem. This enables a patient to have a positive outlook and become less prone to stress acquired from work pressure.[7]

However, there are instances where not all people at work can be so accommodating. There is no specific laboratory exam or x-ray evidence to visibly show the existence of FM once it is diagnosed in a patient. On the outside, patients look fine, but deep inside they are feeling really miserable. Some people are likely to doubt whether the pain is real or if someone who says they are suffering from FM is only claiming to have the disorder. Most patients who choose not to disclose their illness to the people in their workplace may get less consideration from their supervisors and workmates. They may also suffer from bullying and rejection by coworkers. Like most people with disabilities, FM patients are also prone to episodes of rage or anger. This is likely due to the fact that they are experiencing anxiety and social pressure that leads them to reduce social contact with the people around them. This can become a problem at work as it may affect relationships with coworkers, clients, and supervisors.[8]

MANAGING A TIGHT WORK SCHEDULE WITH FIBROMYALGIA

For most, the question of whether they should go to work or not is not really that big of a query. For people suffering from FM, it is not a question of should or should not, it is more of a question of can or cannot. Oftentimes people working their chosen jobs take pleasure in carrying out the physical, social, and intellectual challenges that their careers can bring. Having to deal with FM can add negatively to this list of challenges. At present, more than four million people who suffer from FM remain active in the workforce. Clearly this shows that occupational coping skills can help those who have FM to still be able to stay active and be productive at work. It is possible to stay healthy in order to be able to keep a career on track and garner a steady flow of income. Each case and experience with FM is different for patients who are working professionals, and each workplace is unique in its own way. There are different coping strategies that can be applied to make the workplace more conducive for FM patients.[9]

BE HONEST ABOUT HAVING FM

When suffering from a chronic but relatively uncommon condition, patients sometimes tend to feel ashamed of it. Initially, people conceal the disorder from their employers and coworkers. This is where possible problems may arise. If work colleagues are not entirely aware of the reason why an employee is not able to meet the demands of the job due to fatigue or absences due to frequent medical appointments, the work colleagues may perceive the absent party to be an unreliable employee. Therefore, people suffering from FM should not be afraid to fully disclose to their colleagues that they suffer from FM. It would also be good to explain to them how FM affects a person during the onset of the symptoms, tell them how it affects them, what people surrounding the patient can do to help, and make sure to emphasize to them that it will not affect workflow. Patients can feel overwhelmed and stressed with FM, and when emotions such as resentment, anger, and frustration over having incessant pain arises, productive communication can be hindered. Having an open and honest communication between employers and coworkers about the disorder and its symptoms helps mollify conflicts due to misunderstanding. Patients can also talk to their employers about working out a flexible schedule that allows for adjusted hours to optimize peak production time. For example, if a patient has fewer symptoms first thing in the morning, an early start time can be worked out. If mornings find the patient experiencing more symptoms, then a late start time can be arranged.[10]

OBSERVE SYMPTOMS AND PREPARE IN ADVANCE

Each person has a different set of triggers for different FM symptoms. By scrutinizing the body and taking note of situations that spark the pain, patients can then prepare a plan of action when faced with them. Reading up on pain-management methods that can be applied such as meditating, deep breathing, and biofeedback to help drop chronic pain has proven to be beneficial. Patients who are working professionals may also find it practical to prepare a letter of absence excuse and rehearse a set explanation for whenever they are not feeling well and must tell their colleagues that they are not capable of doing a particular activity at the moment. Another method to try is to keep a weekly work diary and make a schedule of tasks in accordance with the highs and lows of the body's work energy.[11]

Morning persons tend to be more energetic during the daytime, so making sure to focus on the more critical tasks during that time of the day would be most preferable. Likewise, schedule the tasks that are deemed to be of lower priority and are easily accomplished during the afternoon or during the time of day when the patient normally has lower energy. The FM sufferer should always remember to schedule periodic breaks to avoid burnout or stress. Stress and pressure can trigger FM, so it is always best to be able to complete a task as early as possible to avoid hectic, last-minute cramming. Nevertheless, it is also important to recognize that all schedules may not always go as smoothly as planned. There will be situations when FM will be disabling. During those times it is best to reschedule instead of coercing the body to do more than it is able to and ending up having more painful FM flares as a result.[12]

RESTRUCTURE THE WORK AREA

Working on a task that involves a repetitive motion can prove to be even more troubling for those suffering from FM. As much as possible, it is best to be comfortable in the workplace when doing repetitive tasks. Another method of managing FM symptoms in the workplace is by analyzing the workstation and rustling up the necessary changes by taking away anything that might cause any discomfort or might trigger symptoms. Even minor rearrangements such as putting the penholder closer to hand can make a big difference. If a job requires a lot of standing for a long time, reduce leg strain and foot cramps by wearing the proper shoes. A cushioned floor pad can also come in handy to reduce discomfort on the feet. In contrast, if a job entails sitting behind the desk for most of the day, take time to stretch or even stand up from time to time to reduce discomfort. Headaches can occur from eyestrain from looking at a bright laptop or PC screen monitor for a long period of time. Adjust the monitor's brightness to suit the light in the work area, as this will lessen eyestrain and in effect extenuate the probability of getting an annoying headache.[13]

TAKE NOTES OR WRITE A MEMO

To be able to keep a part-time or full-time job, it is necessary to stay not only physically able but also mentally able to manage the job responsibilities. It is a given that when suffering from FM, sleeplessness or medications will sometimes cause brain fog. Whenever possible, the patient can in advance create written instructions or a list of things to do in order to avoid forgetting important assignments or meeting schedules. It is best not to list too much to do in a day. The idea is to set clear and achievable lists of tasks that do not lead to overworking. Seeing a rudimentary roster of things to do will only lead to frustration or disappointment and added stress. It is important to minimize tension. Anxiousness, nervousness, and panic can also cause a flareup of FM symptoms. Doctors have observed that when FM patients are able to control and besiege the pressure in their daily working lives, they also are able to experience less depression, bodily fatigue, and anxiety. Patients are found to be able to sleep better and are able to relax their minds. Because the patients feel that they are in control of their schedule and over their symptoms, FM flares occur less often, and their outlook and quality of life shows great improvement.[14]

ACCEPTING LIMITS

Always keep in mind that even people who are perfectly healthy have personal limits. When FM flares seem unbearable, pause from whatever task is being done and rest. Fibromyalgia patients should learn to decline workloads that are overburdening. Piling on too many commitments will only increase an already heightened stress level and elevate FM pain. Individuals with FM should manage time to do each task properly and follow a daily to-do list that does not necessitate overworking. If health issues such as FM are making it impossible to complete any work assigned from a current job, one should be proactive and think about seeking a different job that will be a better fit. By self-managing the symptoms of FM and controlling daily stress, most people with FM can perform almost anything that a person without the disorder can. Even physical pain that is directly related to work is wieldy through simple adjustments in the workplace that allow patients to continue their vocation.[15]

17

CONCLUSION

In the closing few analyses, FM patients and caregivers should note that exercise, a good sleep routine, and a healthy diet can improve their overall condition. If a person already has concerns with regard to healthy living even before being diagnosed with FM, improving these three areas may be difficult. Sometimes a patient gives into the pain and other FM symptoms rather than trying arduously to see beyond the pain, fatigue, and all the other symptoms associated with an FM diagnosis. It is much better to aim for a healthier lifestyle to improve overall well-being.[1]

GENTLE AND MINDFUL EXERCISE CAN HELP

Although pain and fatigue may fetter the patient from doing some form of exercise, all efforts must be made to start with at least short walks or other gentle exercise as this will have a long-term effect on the improvement of FM symptoms. Yoga can be a good form of exercise for people with FM because it is not strenuous. There may be some difficulty with yoga because of joint and muscle pains, so the patient must take care to select the poses and stretches that are comfortable. In addition, exercise is somewhat for the brain as it releases serotonin, a mood-enhancing chemical. Exercise therefore will be a big help if the patient feels the stress often associated with FM. Another benefit of exercising is that it may fight depression, another symptom that most FM patients also suffer from.[2]

A RESTFUL NIGHT IS A MUST

The body needs a good night's sleep to recuperate from the day, but an FM patient may have restless sleep due to pain. Although a doctor can prescribe medication to help deal with nervy nights and induce sleep, there are alternatives the patient can follow to improve sleep comfort and be more at ease. As mentioned, exercising can be beneficial mainly because exercise stimulates the release of serotonin, which helps normalize an individual's sleep pattern. The patient should avoid exercise within three hours of bedtime because this can lead to wakefulness until the wee hours of the morning. Short afternoon naps are passable, but long daytime naps should be avoided as this might affect the patient's regular sleeping schedule.[3]

Patients with FM are advised to create a dark, sufficiently cool, and quiet environment to make the bedroom more pragmatic for sleep. Aside from the all-important bedroom atmosphere, the person should avoid caffeine and other stimulants before bedtime. The patient should consider soaking in a tub to relax sore muscles and joints or get a massage to feel poised before going to sleep.[4]

EATING HEALTHY IS THE WAY TO GO

Having a healthy diet is important to FM patients as this will provide improved energy levels and overall health. Although there are no specific diets recommended for FM patients, it is best to eat foods that can provide energy. Patients should avoid prepackaged foods because they usually contain ingredients that trigger or worsen FM symptoms. For example, physicians have observed that in some patients, monosodium glutamate (MSG) fuelled the symptoms of FM. Although this is not true in all cases, avoidance of any identified trigger foods is always a better choice. Caffeine may be a culprit too because it can retrogress patients' incidence of migraine and unsettle sleep patterns.[5]

In general, FM patients should devote more time to themselves so that they can take better care of their own well-being. After all, a healthier lifestyle is always a superb way to deal with all diseases. The patient must evaluate which exercise, sleeping tips, and diet works best because the symptoms can vary significantly from one patient to another. Likewise, tips or tasks to counter the symptoms may also differ significantly. Of course, this is easier said than done because even people without a FM diagnosis can find it difficult to live a healthy lifestyle. Still, FM patients must strive to do their best to arrive at the healthiest lifestyle possible. As the old cliché says, health is wealth, and this applies even if one is suffering from a disease that affects the normality of a daily routine. A healthier lifestyle should always be the first approach to conquering any disease, and all FM patients will greatly benefit from following this suggestion.[6]

FINDING MOTIVATION

Since fibromyalgia is a chronic condition, there is the likelihood that it will persist for a long time. It is understandable that dealing with a disease that involves a significant amount of pain and fatigue is not easy. Although it is not life threatening, FM remains a condition that commands consideration from others and motivation for the afflicted in order to cope. While it is common for patients to be taciturn about the disease out of fear of being ostracized because of it, it is a good idea to at least try to set off a dialogue with family, friends, and coworkers so they can understand and accept the patient's diagnosis and offer support when needed.[7]

Support from family members is essential to the life of the person suffering from FM. Understanding the disease should not only be the concern of the patient with the diagnosis but should also be a concern of the family members. If the family is concerned, the relative who suffers from FM will be more motivated to explore ways to reduce the physical and psychological effects of the symptoms. The affected individual must also fully accept the condition in order to find the motivation needed to achieve better well-being. This may only be possible if the diagnosis is also putative among loved ones. Still, even when family members play an important part in the FM course of action, it is up to the patient to move forward without having to constantly rely on other people. Patients must avoid self-pity; they should look for positive things in life that may serve as a motivation to fight or counter the disease.[8]

Consulting medical practitioners and specialists to hunt for answers, advice, and suggestions is also helpful as this can empower the patient. Once the patient feels emboldened, it is easier to conquer the disease and have an easier time adjusting to a new lifestyle. Besides, it is never advisable to keep reticent about the disease because being silent may only worsen the symptoms. It may even stress the patient, which can also lead to increased symptoms. Hence, medical practitioners can be a good source of support and motivation as they can respond to questions and calm the patients' flummoxed emotions.[9]

Community support groups are also a good idea. The support groups can consist of FM patients and others who have loved ones who are suffering from the disorder. This way, everyone in the support group can have a wider perspective in terms of how to deal with the disease. Naturally, it is best to be able to communicate with people who share the experience of the diagnosis, and that is why joining groups that talk about FM is advisable. People can share ideas on how they have coped and dealt with the disease as well as touch others with their own personal chronicles of pain and triumph so that everyone in the group can recognize that they are not the only ones dealing with FM-related tribulations. Furthermore, these groups can show others that they have someone to turn to during their difficult time, as others who have already accepted the reality of the disease can help the newly diagnosed patient understand what to expect from FM and the associated symptoms.[10]

To reiterate, a good support system for one who has FM goes a long way in helping the patient find balance and motivation to go on with life as normally as possible. Things will be different for the patient, and pain will remain a slice of their daily life, but with enough motivation the patient can look beyond the pain and go about life at a new normal—as someone with a FM diagnosis. With motivation from a support group and loved ones, a patient can cultivate the patience to deal with the painful symptoms of the disorder. As already laid out, motivation can be hard to find by trying to solve or accept the changes alone. It is always good to have the support of others because then changes are easier to bear.[11]

PATIENCE IS KEY

Experiencing pain and fatigue all throughout life is never easy. It can be physically, emotionally, and psychologically wearisome to go through all the pain that comes with the disease on a daily basis. Because of this, patience is very crucial when dealing with FM, and it is essential when preparing to make lifestyle changes for a downturn of symptoms. A patient may have to stop engaging in activities that were once enjoyable but that can no longer be done because of the symptoms of the disease. Patients must be careful when doing certain activities even if they are of a light nature because they might cause discomfort.[12]

Likewise, since there are no specific tests to determine FM, the patient must undergo a battery of tests in order for the doctor to determine if FM is the correct diagnosis. Repetitive tests can be irritating, so patience will really be a virtue during this period.[13]

Memory loss is also a common symptom of FM, so the patient must have patience when faced with the inability to recollect. The FM sufferer must have the patience to jot down notes to help remember appointments or other tasks that must be accomplished. The family of an FM patient must also apply patience because of the affected person's memory loss. Certain tasks would have to be delegated to other family members because the patient may become unable to perform the particular tasks.[14]

In terms of employment, some patients may have to look for a new job if their current one no longer suits them and cannot be adapted to accommodate the FM symptoms and limitations. This is because they may not be able to perform their workload anymore. This drastic change in employment validates the idea that patience is indeed vital when dealing with FM. Naturally, it is unnecessary to herald to the whole world that a person has been diagnosed with FM, but it could be helpful if the company management knows about the diagnosis so they can help with adapting schedules or tasks. This could possibly lead to job reassignment. In the event that the managers or supervisors cannot accept the parameters of the condition, the patient will have to look for other employment. Fibromyalgia does not mean that the patient can no longer work, it just means there are considerations to be made on the part of both the employee and the employer.[15]

If the patient was physically active before being diagnosed and no longer has the capacity to be as active as prior to the development of symptoms, the patient may experience frustration or depression. Even family members may have to alter their lifestyle and their day-to-day activities to accommodate the sine qua non of the person with the diagnosis. Whichever way an individual patient's story goes, everyone involved will have to be a little bit more patient with each other.[16]

Since FM is a trial and elimination disease, the patient must put up with all its complexities. Things will really be different for the person who has FM, but the patient must not give up on life because of a diagnosis. Once the patient gets into the routine of the adjustments necessary to counter the symptoms of FM, life will improve and every-one's patience will have paid off.[17]

Again, with all of the changes that an FM patient has to make, patience is very important and will always be key to dealing with and accepting the condition. If family members do not have the patience to accept the condition, the patient may pull out and feel emotionally low, thereby worsening the situation and encountering depression. This would make matters worse not only for the patient but also for the whole family. A stressful environment could develop, and it would do nothing but have a vile impression on the person with FM.[18]

THE IMPORTANCE OF CONSULTING A DOCTOR

There is no specific test to determine FM. Doctors usually do a series of evaluations to surmise whether the patient does indeed have FM. Therefore, it is important to consult a doctor so a precise diagnosis can be made, particularly because the disease shares symptoms with other disorders. One might have to consult with more than one physician to be sure that the diagnosis is actually FM. A second opinion or consulta-tion with a specialist might be required.[19]

A patient needs proper advice on how to stifle the effects of FM symptoms to at least be comfortable. Since there is no single medica-tion to treat all of the known FM symptoms, it is important to have the proper medications for pain, insomnia, or depression that patients are likely to undergo as part of the disease. However, since some patients may develop allergies or have adverse reactions to prescribed medicine, it is important to be tested for sensitivity to a drug.[20]

The whole ball of wax known about FM points to one thing: It is always focal to consult a doctor for a proper diagnosis first because the patient may have questions about the disease. Furthermore, medical practitioners who specialize in FM are adroit individuals who offer advice, prescribe medication, and develop other treatment schemes in order to rout symptoms. Doctors can also provide exhortation on the various types of food that can trigger some of the symptoms of the disorder. They can also recommend exercises and other activities that can make the patient feel better. They know which medication would work best for which symptom.[21]

Doing things or handling symptoms without consulting a doctor is a major recipe for disaster. Even patients who regularly go online to read more about the disease still need medical doctors to help them become more educated about their individual cases. Doing research so that one can formulate questions to ask the doctor during a consultation is a good idea, but collaring symptoms and treatments without consulting a doctor can result in adverse effects, including new or worsened symptoms.[22]

Yes, some people may become stressed when they hear that they need to go to the doctor. This should not be the case, though, because consulting with someone who is familiar with FM can lead to improved health and well-being. People may take the disease for granted and accept that life will forever include symptoms such as pain, depression, and sleeplessness when consulting someone well versed in the field can bring about a better prognosis. Wrong presumptions may lead to more complications, which may lead to more health trepidations for the person whose FM remains undiagnosed. Since it is the duty of a doctor to make accurate findings in order to help people manage their symptoms, a patient should allow a doctor the opportunity to help alleviate symptoms.[23]

While FM is not a curable disease, its symptoms are attenuated with healthier lifestyle choices. As a final note, after a FM diagnosis, patients must fully assent to the fact they have the disease for them to make the necessary changes to cope with it.[24]

NOTES

PREFACE

1. Simons DG. Traumatic fibromyositis or myofascial trigger points? West J Med. 1978 Jan;128(1):69–71.

2. Borg-Stein J, Stein J. Trigger points and tender points: one and the same? Does injection treatment help? Rheum Dis Clin North Am. 1996 May;22(2):305–22.

3. Goldenberg DL. Diagnosis and differential diagnosis of fibromyalgia. Am J Med. 2009 Dec;122(12 Suppl):S14–21.

4. Arnold LM, Clauw DJ, McCarberg BH; FibroCollaborative. Improving the recognition and diagnosis of fibromyalgia. Mayo Clin Proc. 2011 May;86(5):457–64.

5. Staud R. Treatment of fibromyalgia and its symptoms. Expert Opin Pharmacother. 2007 Aug;8(11):1629–42.

6. Bernard AL, Prince A, Edsall P. Quality of life issues for fibromyalgia patients. Arthritis Care Res. 2000 Feb;13(1):42–50.

7. Burckhardt CS, Bjelle A. Education programmes for fibromyalgia patients: description and evaluation. Baillieres Clin Rheumatol. 1994 Nov;8(4):935–55.

8. Hsu MC, Schubiner H, Lumley MA, Stracks JS, Clauw DJ, Williams DA. Sustained pain reduction through affective self-awareness in fibromyalgia: a randomized controlled trial. J Gen Intern Med. 2010 Oct;25(10):1064–70.

1. HISTORY OF FIBROMYALGIA

1. Luo JJ, Dun N. Chronic pain: myofascial pain and fibromyalgia. Int J Phys Med Rehabil. 2013 Aug 5;(1):e102.

2. Bjelle A, Bengtsson A, Henriksson KG, Idström JP, Torebjörk E, Thornell LE. [Fibromyalgia: a new name for a syndrome with diffuse muscular disorders]. Lakartidningen. 1989 Feb 15;86(7):528–30.

3. Roxberg A, Sameby J, Brodin S, Fridlund B, da Silva AB. Out of the wave: the meaning of suffering and relief from suffering as described in auto-biographies by survivors of the 2004 Indian Ocean tsunami. Int J Qual Stud Health Well-Being. 2010 Oct 14;5(3).

4. Bubnov RV. Evidence-based pain management: is the concept of inte-grative medicine applicable? EPMA J. 2012 Oct 22;3(1):13; Apuzzo D, Giotti C, Pasqualetti P, Ferrazza P, Soldati P, Zucco GM. An observational retrospec-tive/horizontal study to compare oxygen-ozone therapy and/or global postural re-education in complicated chronic low back pain. Funct Neurol. 2014 Jan–Mar;29(1):31–9.

5. Schäfer ML. [On the history of the concept neurasthenia and its mod-ern variants chronic-fatigue-syndrome, fibromyalgia and multiple chemical sensitivities]. Fortschr Neurol Psychiatr. 2002 Nov;70(11):570–82.

6. Bennett RM. Fibrositis: misnomer for a common rheumatic disorder. West J Med. 1981 May;134(5):405–13.

7. Chandola HC, Chakraborty A. Fibromyalgia and myofascial pain syn-drome—a dilemma. Indian J Anaesth. 2009 Oct;53(5):575–81; Simons DG. Fibrositis/fibromyalgia: a form of myofascial trigger points? Am J Med. 1986 Sep 29;81(3A):93–98.

8. Hunder GG, Matteson EL. Rheumatology practice at Mayo Clinic: the first 40 years—1920 to 1960. Mayo Clin Proc. 2010 Apr;85(4):e17–30.

9. Halliday JL. The psychological approach to rheumatism: (section of physical medicine). Proc R Soc Med. 1938 Jan;31(3):167–178.2.

10. Duthie JJR. Arthritis and allied conditions. A textbook of rheumatology. Ann Rheum Dis. 1973 Jul;32(4):394–95.

11. Traut EF. Fibrositis. J Am Geriatr Soc. 1968 May;16(5):531–38.

12. Chandola HC, Chakraborty A. Fibromyalgia and myofascial pain syn-drome—a dilemma. Indian J Anaesth. 2009 Oct;53(5):575–81; Bellato E, Mari-ni E, Castoldi F, Barbasetti N, Mattei L, Bonasia DE, Blonna D. Fibromyalgia syndrome: etiology, pathogenesis, diagnosis, and treatment. Pain Res Treat. 2012;2012:426130.

13. Fitzcharles MA, Yunus MB. The clinical concept of fibromyalgia as a changing paradigm in the past 20 years. Pain Res Treat. 2012;2012:184835.

14. Moret C, Briley M. Antidepressants in the treatment of fibromyalgia. Neuropsychiatr Dis Treat. 2006 Dec;2(4):537–48.

15. Yunus MB. The prevalence of fibromyalgia in other chronic pain conditions. Pain Res Treat. 2012;2012:584573.

16. Wolfe F, Cathey MA, Kleinheksel SM. Fibrositis (Fibromyalgia) in rheumatoid arthritis. J Rheumatol. 1984 Dec;11(6):814–18.

17. Burckhardt CS, Clark SR, Bennett RM. The fibromyalgia impact questionnaire: development and validation. J Rheumatol. 1991 May;18(5):728–33.

18. Granges G, Littlejohn GO. A comparative study of clinical signs in fibromyalgia/fibrositis syndrome, healthy and exercising subjects. J Rheumatol. 1993 Feb;20(2):344–51.

19. Buskila D, Sarzi-Puttini P. Biology and therapy of fibromyalgia. Genetic aspects of fibromyalgia syndrome. Arthritis Res Ther. 2006 Jul;8(5):218.

20. Carette S, Bell MJ, Reynolds WJ, Haraoui B, McCain GA, Bykerk VP, Edworthy SM, Baron M, Koehler BE, Fam AG, et al. Comparison of amitriptyline, cyclobenzaprine, and placebo in the treatment of fibromyalgia. A randomized, double-blind clinical trial. Arthritis Rheum. 1994 Jan;37(1):32–40; Moret C, Briley M. Antidepressants in the treatment of fibromyalgia. Neuropsychiatr Dis Treat. 2006 Dec;2(4):537–48.

21. Galek A, Erbslöh-Möller B, Köllner V, Kühn-Becker H, Langhorst J, Petermann F, Prothmann U, Winkelmann A, Häuser W. [Mental disorders in patients with fibromyalgia syndrome: screening in centres of different medical specialties]. Schmerz. 2013 Jun;27(3):296–304.

22. [No authors listed]. Understanding fibromyalgia and its related disorders. Prim Care Companion J Clin Psychiatry. 2008;10(2):133–44.

23. Hoffman SJ, Tan C. Biological, psychological and social processes that explain celebrities' influence on patients' health-related behaviors. Arch Public Health. 2015 Jan 19;73(1):3.

24. Chiarella T. This earth that holds me fast will find me breath: the Morgan Freeman story. *Esquire*, July 9, 2012. Accessed August 21, 2015. http://www.esquire.com/entertainment/movies/interviews/a14768/morgan-freeman-interview-0812/.

25. Green W. Numbness, insomnia, constant pain and fatigue . . . just some of the symptoms of a debilitating illness that affects 1.8m Britons. *Daily Mail*, September 17, 2012. Accessed August 29, 2015. http://www.dailymail.co.uk/health/article-2203735/Fibromyalgia-Neurological-condition-causing-numbness-insomnia-pain-fatigue-1-8m-Britons.html.

26. Fowler B. Famous faces of fibromyalgia. *Healthline*, February 27, 2013. Accessed August 29, 2015. http://www.healthline.com/health-slideshow/celebrities-fibromyalgia.

27. Fowler B. Famous faces of fibromyalgia. *Healthline*, February 27, 2013. Accessed August 29, 2015. http://www.healthline.com/health-slideshow/celebrities-fibromyalgia.

28. Fowler B. Famous faces of fibromyalgia. *Healthline*, February 27, 2013. Accessed August 29, 2015. http://www.healthline.com/health-slideshow/celebrities-fibromyalgia.

29. Chase K. Garofalo directs stinging wit toward herself. *Boston Globe* (Boston.com), May 11, 2009. Accessed September 2, 2015. http://www.boston.com/ae/theater_arts/comedy/articles/2009/05/11/garofalo_directs_stinging_wit_toward_herself/.

30. Richards K. 10 Celebrities With Fibromyalgia. February 12, 2014. Accessed September 29, 2015. www.prohealth.com/library/showArticle.cfm?libid=18748.

31. Morgan J. A.J. Langer mellows out to fight fibromyalgia. *USA Today*, April 9, 2001. Accessed September 29, 2015. http://usatoday30.usatoday.com/news/health/spotlight/2001-04-09-langer-fibromyalgia.htm.

32. Fowler B. Famous faces of fibromyalgia. *Healthline*, February 27, 2013. Accessed August 29, 2015. http://www.healthline.com/health-slideshow/celebrities-fibromyalgia.

33. Childers L. Mary McDonough's lessons from a lupus diagnosis: how the "Waltons" star and activist deals with symptoms of lupus. *Lifescript*, March 29, 2012. Accessed September 29, 2015. http://www.lifescript.com/health/centers/lupus/articles/mary_mcdonoughs_lessons_from_a_lupus_diagnosis.aspx.

34. Model Jo Guest: Mystery illness has "ruined my career." *Daily Mail*, January 23, 2008. Accessed September 9, 2015. http://www.dailymail.co.uk/tvshowbiz/article-509554/Model-Jo-Guest-Mystery-illness-ruined-career.html.

35. Clauw DJ. Fibromyalgia: an overview. Am J Med. 2009 Dec;122(12 Suppl):S3–S13.

2. CONNECTIONS BETWEEN FIBROMYALGIA AND CHRONIC FATIGUE SYNDROME

1. Friedberg F. Chronic fatigue syndrome, fibromyalgia, and related illnesses: a clinical model of assessment and intervention. J Clin Psychol. 2010 Jun;66(6):641–65.

2. Jason LA, Taylor RR, Kennedy CL. Chronic fatigue syndrome, fibromyalgia, and multiple chemical sensitivities in a community-based sample of persons with chronic fatigue syndrome-like symptoms. Psychosom Med. 2000 Sep–Oct;62(5):655–63.

3. Van Houdenhove B, Kempke S, Luyten P. Psychiatric aspects of chronic fatigue syndrome and fibromyalgia. Curr Psychiatry Rep. 2010 Jun;12(3):208–14; Friedberg F, Jason LA. Chronic fatigue syndrome and fibromyalgia: clinical assessment and treatment. J Clin Psychol. 2001 Apr;57(4):433–55.

4. Afari N, Buchwald D. Chronic fatigue syndrome: a review. Am J Psychiatry. 2003 Feb;160(2):221–36; Plioplys AV, Plioplys S. Amantadine and L-carnitine treatment of Chronic Fatigue Syndrome. Neuropsychobiology. 1997;35(1):16–23.

5. Clauw DJ. Fibromyalgia: a clinical review. JAMA. 2014 Apr 16;311(15):1547–55.

6. Younger J, Parkitny L, McLain D. The use of low-dose naltrexone (LDN) as a novel anti-inflammatory treatment for chronic pain. Clin Rheumatol. 2014 Apr;33(4):451–59; Stewart RE, Chambless DL. Cognitive-behavioral therapy for adult anxiety disorders in clinical practice: a meta-analysis of effectiveness studies. J Consult Clin Psychol. 2009 Aug;77(4):595–606.

7. Cook DB, Stegner AJ, Nagelkirk PR, Meyer JD, Togo F, Natelson BH. Responses to exercise differ for chronic fatigue syndrome patients with fibromyalgia. Med Sci Sports Exerc. 2012 Jun;44(6):1186–93; Cook DB, Nagelkirk PR, Poluri A, Mores J, Natelson BH. The influence of aerobic fitness and fibromyalgia on cardiorespiratory and perceptual responses to exercise in patients with chronic fatigue syndrome. Arthritis Rheum. 2006 Oct;54(10):3351–62.

8. Lavergne MR, Cole DC, Kerr K, Marshall LM. Functional impairment in chronic fatigue syndrome, fibromyalgia, and multiple chemical sensitivity. Can Fam Physician. 2010 Feb;56(2):e57–65.

9. Aaron LA, Herrell R, Ashton S, Belcourt M, Schmaling K, Goldberg J, Buchwald D. Comorbid clinical conditions in chronic fatigue: a co-twin control study. J Gen Intern Med. 2001 Jan;16(1):24–31.

10. Griffith JP, Zarrouf FA. A systematic review of Chronic Fatigue Syndrome: don't assume it's depression. Prim Care Companion J Clin Psychiatry. 2008;10(2):120–28; Yancey JR, Thomas SM. Chronic fatigue syndrome: diagnosis and treatment. Am Fam Physician. 2012 Oct 15;86(8):741–46.

11. Sharpe M. Non-pharmacological approaches to treatment. Ciba Found Symp. 1993;173:298–308; discussion 308–17.

12. Turner J, Kelly B. Emotional dimensions of chronic disease. West J Med. 2000 Feb;172(2):124–28.

13. Friedberg F, Leung DW, Quick J. Do support groups help people with chronic fatigue syndrome and fibromyalgia? A comparison of active and inactive members. J Rheumatol. 2005 Dec;32(12):2416–20.

14. van Koulil S, Effting M, Kraaimaat FW, van Lankveld W, van Helmond T, Cats H, van Riel PL, de Jong AJ, Haverman JF, Evers AW. Cognitive-behavioural therapies and exercise programmes for patients with fibromyalgia: state of the art and future directions. Ann Rheum Dis. 2007 May;66(5):571–81. Epub 2006 Aug 17.

15. Mease PJ. Further strategies for treating fibromyalgia: the role of serotonin and norepinephrine reuptake inhibitors. Am J Med. 2009 Dec;122(12 Suppl):S44–55; Hsueh HF, Jarrett ME, Cain KC, Burr RL, Deechakawan W, Heitkemper MM. Does a self-management program change dietary intake in adults with irritable bowel syndrome? Gastroenterol Nurs. 2011 Mar–Apr;34(2):108–16.

16. Kishi A, Natelson BH, Togo F, Struzik ZR, Rapoport DM, Yamamoto Y. Sleep stage transitions in chronic fatigue syndrome patients with or without fibromyalgia. Conf Proc IEEE Eng Med Biol Soc. 2010;2010:5391–94.

17. Lavergne MR, Cole DC, Kerr K, Marshall LM. Functional impairment in chronic fatigue syndrome, fibromyalgia, and multiple chemical sensitivity. Can Fam Physician. 2010 Feb;56(2):e57–65.

18. Sumpton JE, Moulin DE. Fibromyalgia: presentation and management with a focus on pharmacological treatment. Pain Res Manag. 2008 Nov–Dec;13(6):477–83.

19. Van Houdenhove B, Neerinckx E, Onghena P, Vingerhoets A, Lysens R, Vertommen H. Daily hassles reported by chronic fatigue syndrome and fibromyalgia patients in tertiary care: a controlled quantitative and qualitative study. Psychother Psychosom. 2002 Jul–Aug;71(4):207–13.

20. Van Houdenhove B, Egle UT. Fibromyalgia: a stress disorder? Piecing the biopsychosocial puzzle together. Psychother Psychosom. 2004 Sep–Oct;73(5):267–75.

21. Van Houdenhove B, Egle UT. Fibromyalgia: a stress disorder? Piecing the biopsychosocial puzzle together. Psychother Psychosom. 2004 Sep–Oct;73(5):267–75.

22. Reynolds KJ, Vernon SD, Bouchery E, Reeves WC. The economic impact of chronic fatigue syndrome. Cost Eff Resour Alloc. 2004 Jun 21;2(1):4.

23. [No authors listed]. Understanding fibromyalgia and its related disorders. Prim Care Companion J Clin Psychiatry. 2008;10(2):133–44.

24. [No authors listed]. Understanding fibromyalgia and its related disorders. Prim Care Companion J Clin Psychiatry. 2008;10(2):133–44.

25. Parrish BP, Zautra AJ, Davis MC. The role of positive and negative interpersonal events on daily fatigue in women with fibromyalgia, rheumatoid arthritis, and osteoarthritis. Health Psychol. 2008 Nov;27(6):694–702.

26. Buchwald D. Fibromyalgia and chronic fatigue syndrome: similarities and differences. Rheum Dis Clin North Am. 1996 May;22(2):219–43; Chia JK.

The role of enterovirus in chronic fatigue syndrome. J Clin Pathol. 2005 Nov;58(11):1126–32.

27. Goldenberg DL. Fibromyalgia and its relation to chronic fatigue syndrome, viral illness and immune abnormalities. J Rheumatol Suppl. 1989 Nov;19:91–93.

28. Parker AJ, Wessely S, Cleare AJ. The neuroendocrinology of Chronic Fatigue Syndrome and fibromyalgia. Psychol Med. 2001 Nov;31(8):1331–45; Tang LW, Zheng H, Chen L, Zhou SY, Huang WJ, Li Y, Wu X. Gray matter volumes in patients with chronic fatigue syndrome. Evid Based Complement Alternat Med. 2015;2015:380615.

29. Friedberg F, Williams DA, Collinge W. Lifestyle-oriented non-pharmacological treatments for fibromyalgia: a clinical overview and applications with home-based technologies. J Pain Res. 2012;5:425–35.

3. HOW BODY SYSTEMS ARE AFFECTED SYMPTOMATICALLY BY FIBROMYALGIA

1. Bellato E, Marini E, Castoldi F, Barbasetti N, Mattei L, Bonasia DE, Blonna D. Fibromyalgia syndrome: etiology, pathogenesis, diagnosis, and treatment. Pain Res Treat. 2012;2012:426130.

2. Cassisi G, Sarzi-Puttini P, Alciati A, Casale R, Bazzichi L, Carignola R, Gracely RH, Salaffi F, Marinangeli F, Torta R, Giamberardino MA, Buskila D, Spath M, Cazzola M, Di Franco M, Biasi G, Stisi S, Altomonte L, Arioli G, Leardini G, Gorla R, Marsico A, Ceccherelli F, Atzeni F; Italian Fibromyalgia Network. Symptoms and signs in fibromyalgia syndrome. Reumatismo. 2008 Jul–Sep;60 Suppl 1:15–24.

3. Gupta A, Silman AJ. Psychological stress and fibromyalgia: a review of the evidence suggesting a neuroendocrine link. Arthritis Res Ther. 2004;6(3):98–106.

4. Petersel DL, Dror V, Cheung R. Central amplification and fibromyalgia: disorder of pain processing. J Neurosci Res. 2011 Jan;89(1):29–34.

5. Watson NF, Buchwald D, Goldberg J, Noonan C, Ellenbogen RG. Neurologic signs and symptoms in fibromyalgia. Arthritis Rheum. 2009 Sep;60(9):2839–44.

6. Schmidt-Wilcke T, Kairys A, Ichesco E, Fernandez-Sanchez ML, Barjola P, Heitzeg M, Harris RE, Clauw DJ, Glass J, Williams DA. Changes in clinical pain in fibromyalgia patients correlate with changes in brain activation in the cingulate cortex in a response inhibition task. Pain Med. 2014 Aug;15(8):1346–58.

7. Rhodus NL, Fricton J, Carlson P, Messner R. Oral symptoms associated with fibromyalgia syndrome. J Rheumatol. 2003 Aug;30(8):1841–45.

8. Stray LL, Kristensen Ø, Lomeland M, Skorstad M, Stray T, Tønnessen FE. Motor regulation problems and pain in adults diagnosed with ADHD. Behav Brain Funct. 2013 May 3;9:18.

9. Sumpton JE, Moulin DE. Fibromyalgia: presentation and management with a focus on pharmacological treatment. Pain Res Manag. 2008 Nov–Dec;13(6):477–83.

10. Leavitt F, Katz RS, Mills M, Heard AR. Cognitive and dissociative manifestations in fibromyalgia. J Clin Rheumatol. 2002 Apr;8(2):77–84.

11. Muto LH, Sauer JF, Yuan SL, Sousa A, Mango PC, Marques AP. Postural control and balance self-efficacy in women with fibromyalgia: are there differences? Eur J Phys Rehabil Med. 2015 Apr;51(2):149–54.

12. Spaeth M, Rizzi M, Sarzi-Puttini P. Fibromyalgia and sleep. Best Pract Res Clin Rheumatol. 2011 Apr;25(2):227–39.

13. Watson NF, Buchwald D, Goldberg J, Noonan C, Ellenbogen RG. Neurologic signs and symptoms in fibromyalgia. Arthritis Rheum. 2009 Sep;60(9):2839–44; Bäckman E, Bengtsson A, Bengtsson M, Lennmarken C, Henriksson KG. Skeletal muscle function in primary fibromyalgia. Effect of regional sympathetic blockade with guanethidine. Acta Neurol Scand. 1988 Mar;77(3):187–91.

14. Bäckman E, Bengtsson A, Bengtsson M, Lennmarken C, Henriksson KG. Skeletal muscle function in primary fibromyalgia. Effect of regional sympathetic blockade with guanethidine. Acta Neurol Scand. 1988 Mar;77(3):187–91.

15. Henriksson KG. Fibromyalgia—from syndrome to disease. Overview of pathogenetic mechanisms. J Rehabil Med. 2003 May;(41 Suppl):89–94.

16. Chandola HC, Chakraborty A. Fibromyalgia and myofascial pain syndrome—a dilemma. Indian J Anaesth. 2009 Oct;53(5):575–81.

17. Lipton RB, Bigal ME, Steiner TJ, Silberstein SD, Olesen J. Classification of primary headaches. Neurology. 2004 Aug 10;63(3):427–35; Peres MF. Fibromyalgia, fatigue, and headache disorders. Curr Neurol Neurosci Rep. 2003 Mar;3(2):97–103; de Tommaso M, Federici A, Serpino C, Vecchio E, Franco G, Sardaro M, Delussi M, Livrea P. Clinical features of headache patients with fibromyalgia comorbidity. J Headache Pain. 2011 Dec;12(6):629–38.

18. Vincent A, Benzo RP, Whipple MO, McAllister SJ, Erwin PJ, Saligan LN. Beyond pain in fibromyalgia: insights into the symptom of fatigue. Arthritis Res Ther. 2013;15(6):221; Casale R, Rainoldi A. Fatigue and fibromyalgia syndrome: clinical and neurophysiologic pattern. Best Pract Res Clin Rheumatol. 2011 Apr;25(2):241–47.

19. Abdullah M, Vishwanath S, Elbalkhi A, Ambrus JL Jr. Mitochondrial myopathy presenting as fibromyalgia: a case report. J Med Case Rep. 2012 Feb 10;6:55.

20. Calandre EP, Vilchez JS, Molina-Barea R, Tovar MI, Garcia-Leiva JM, Hidalgo J, Rodriguez-Lopez CM, Rico-Villademoros F. Suicide attempts and risk of suicide in patients with fibromyalgia: a survey in Spanish patients. Rheumatology (Oxford). 2011 Oct;50(10):1889–93.

21. Lurie M, Caidahl K, Johansson G, Bake B. Respiratory function in chronic primary fibromyalgia. Scand J Rehabil Med. 1990;22(3):151–55.

22. Pamuk ON, Umit H, Harmandar O. Increased frequency of gastrointestinal symptoms in patients with fibromyalgia and associated factors: a comparative study. J Rheumatol. 2009 Aug;36(8):1720–24.

23. Arnold LM, Clauw DJ, Dunegan LJ, Turk DC; FibroCollaborative. A framework for fibromyalgia management for primary care providers. Mayo Clin Proc. 2012 May;87(5):488–96.

24. Bellato E, Marini E, Castoldi F, Barbasetti N, Mattei L, Bonasia DE, Blonna D. Fibromyalgia syndrome: etiology, pathogenesis, diagnosis, and treatment. Pain Res Treat. 2012;2012:426130.

4. BRAIN FOG: MYTH OR REALITY?

1. Ocon AJ. Caught in the thickness of brain fog: exploring the cognitive symptoms of Chronic Fatigue Syndrome. Front Physiol. 2013 Apr 5;4:63; Theoharides TC, Zhang B. Neuro-inflammation, blood-brain barrier, seizures and autism. J Neuroinflammation. 2011 Nov 30;8:168.

2. Kravitz HM, Katz RS. Fibrofog and fibromyalgia: a narrative review and implications for clinical practice. Rheumatol Int. 2015 Jul;35(7):1115–25.

3. Erecińska M, Silver IA. ATP and brain function. J Cereb Blood Flow Metab. 1989 Feb;9(1):2–19.

4. Markou A, Duka T, Prelevic GM. Estrogens and brain function. Hormones (Athens). 2005 Jan–Mar;4(1):9–17; Ross AJ, Medow MS, Rowe PC, Stewart JM. What is brain fog? An evaluation of the symptom in postural tachycardia syndrome. Clin Auton Res. 2013 Dec;23(6):305–11.

5. Strauchman M, Morningstar MW. Fluoroquinolone toxicity symptoms in a patient presenting with low back pain. Clin Pract. 2012 Nov 28;2(4):e87; Medlin J. Environmental toxins and the brain. Environ Health Perspect. 1996 Aug;104(8):822–23.

6. Bremner JD. Traumatic stress: effects on the brain. Dialogues Clin Neurosci. 2006 Dec;8(4):445–61; Ocon AJ. Caught in the thickness of brain

fog: exploring the cognitive symptoms of Chronic Fatigue Syndrome. Front Physiol. 2013 Apr 5;4:63.

7. Medina KL, Schweinsburg AD, Cohen-Zion M, Nagel BJ, Tapert SF. Effects of alcohol and combined marijuana and alcohol use during adolescence on hippocampal volume and asymmetry. Neurotoxicol Teratol. 2007 Jan–Feb;29(1):141–52. Epub 2006 Dec 12; Ocon AJ. Caught in the thickness of brain fog: exploring the cognitive symptoms of Chronic Fatigue Syndrome. Front Physiol. 2013 Apr 5;4:63.

8. Kravitz HM, Katz RS. Fibrofog and fibromyalgia: a narrative review and implications for clinical practice. Rheumatol Int. 2015 Jul;35(7):1115–25; Theoharides TC, Stewart JM, Panagiotidou S, Melamed I. Mast cells, brain inflammation and autism. Eur J Pharmacol. 2015 May 1. pii: S0014–2999(15)00398-2.

9. Shanks L, Jason LA, Evans M, Brown A. Cognitive impairments associated with CFS and POTS. Front Physiol. 2013 May 16;4:113.

10. Ross AJ, Medow MS, Rowe PC, Stewart JM. What is brain fog? An evaluation of the symptom in postural tachycardia syndrome. Clin Auton Res. 2013 Dec;23(6):305–11.

11. Etnier JL, Karper WB, Gapin JI, Barella LA, Chang YK, Murphy KJ. Exercise, fibromyalgia, and fibrofog: a pilot study. J Phys Act Health. 2009 Mar;6(2):239–46.

12. Gómez-Pinilla F. Brain foods: the effects of nutrients on brain function. Nat Rev Neurosci. 2008 Jul;9(7):568–78; Benington JH, Heller HC. Restoration of brain energy metabolism as the function of sleep. Prog Neurobiol. 1995 Mar;45(4):347–60.

13. Glass JM. Review of cognitive dysfunction in fibromyalgia: a convergence on working memory and attentional control impairments. Rheum Dis Clin North Am. 2009 May;35(2):299–311; Maes M, Libbrecht I, Van Hunsel F, Lin AH, De Clerck L, Stevens W, Kenis G, de Jongh R, Bosmans E, Neels H. The immune-inflammatory pathophysiology of fibromyalgia: increased serum soluble gp130, the common signal transducer protein of various neurotrophic cytokines. Psychoneuroendocrinology. 1999 May;24(4):371–83.

14. Gillett G. Medical science, culture, and truth. Philos Ethics Humanit Med. 2006 Dec 19;1:13.

15. Alderson P. The importance of theories in health care. BMJ. 1998 Oct 10;317(7164):1007–10.

16. Kravitz HM, Katz RS. Fibrofog and fibromyalgia: a narrative review and implications for clinical practice. Rheumatol Int. 2015 Jul;35(7):1115–25.

5. CAUSES OF FIBROMYALGIA

1. Sandstrom MJ, Keefe FJ. Self-management of fibromyalgia: the role of formal coping skills training and physical exercise training programs. Arthritis Care Res. 1998 Dec;11(6):432–47.

2. Offenbächer M, Stucki G. Physical therapy in the treatment of fibromyalgia. Scand J Rheumatol Suppl. 2000;113:78–85.

3. Neumann L, Buskila D. Epidemiology of fibromyalgia. Curr Pain Headache Rep. 2003 Oct;7(5):362–68.

4. Usui C, Hatta K, Aratani S, Yagishita N, Nishioka K, Okamura S, Itoh K, Yamano Y, Nakamura H, Asukai N, Nakajima T, Nishioka K. Vulnerability to traumatic stress in fibromyalgia patients: 19 month follow-up after the great East Japan disaster. Arthritis Res Ther. 2013 Sep 23;15(5):R130.

5. Bernik M, Sampaio TP, Gandarela L. Fibromyalgia comorbid with anxiety disorders and depression: combined medical and psychological treatment. Curr Pain Headache Rep. 2013 Sep;17(9):358.

6. Tyrer P, Baldwin D. Generalised anxiety disorder. Lancet. 2006 Dec 16;368(9553):2156–66.

7. Heidari Gorji MA, Davanloo AA, Heidarigorji AM. The efficacy of relaxation training on stress, anxiety, and pain perception in hemodialysis patients. Indian J Nephrol. 2014 Nov–Dec;24(6):356–61.

8. Jensen KB, Petzke F, Carville S, Fransson P, Marcus H, Williams SC, Choy E, Mainguy Y, Gracely R, Ingvar M, Kosek E. Anxiety and depressive symptoms in fibromyalgia are related to poor perception of health but not to pain sensitivity or cerebral processing of pain. Arthritis Rheum. 2010 Nov;62(11):3488–95; Johnson LM, Zautra AJ, Davis MC. The role of illness uncertainty on coping with fibromyalgia symptoms. Health Psychol. 2006 Nov;25(6):696–703.

9. Meeus M, Nijs J, Vanderheiden T, Baert I, Descheemaeker F, Struyf F. The effect of relaxation therapy on autonomic functioning, symptoms and daily functioning, in patients with chronic fatigue syndrome or fibromyalgia: a systematic review. Clin Rehabil. 2015 Mar;29(3):221–33.

10. Kurtze N, Gundersen KT, Svebak S. Quality of life, functional disability and lifestyle among subgroups of fibromyalgia patients: the significance of anxiety and depression. Br J Med Psychol. 1999 Dec;72 (Pt 4):471–84.

11. Picard P, Jusseaume C, Boutet M, Dualé C, Mulliez A, Aublet-Cuvellier B. Hypnosis for management of fibromyalgia. Int J Clin Exp Hypn. 2013;61(1):111–23.

12. Van Houdenhove B, Egle U, Luyten P. The role of life stress in fibromyalgia. Curr Rheumatol Rep. 2005 Oct;7(5):365–70.

13. Schmidt S, Grossman P, Schwarzer B, Jena S, Naumann J, Walach H. Treating fibromyalgia with mindfulness-based stress reduction: results from a 3-armed randomized controlled trial. Pain. 2011 Feb;152(2):361–69.

14. Ruiz-Pérez I, Plazaola-Castaño J, Cáliz-Cáliz R, Rodríguez-Calvo I, García-Sánchez A, Ferrer-González MA, Guzmán-Ubeda M, del Río-Lozano M, López-Chicheri García I. Risk factors for fibromyalgia: the role of violence against women. Clin Rheumatol. 2009 Jul;28(7):777–86.

15. Winfield JB. Psychological determinants of fibromyalgia and related syndromes. Curr Rev Pain. 2000;4(4):276–86; Ruiz-Pérez I, Plazaola-Castaño J, Cáliz-Cáliz R, Rodríguez-Calvo I, García-Sánchez A, Ferrer-González MA, Guzmán-Ubeda M, del Río-Lozano M, López-Chicheri García I. Risk factors for fibromyalgia: the role of violence against women. Clin Rheumatol. 2009 Jul;28(7):777–86.

16. Friedberg F, Williams DA, Collinge W. Lifestyle-oriented non-pharmacological treatments for fibromyalgia: a clinical overview and applications with home-based technologies. J Pain Res. 2012;5:425–35.

6. OUTPATIENT VS. INPATIENT CARE IN FIBROMYALGIA TREATMENT

1. Bennett RM, Burckhardt CS, Clark SR, O'Reilly CA, Wiens AN, Campbell SM. Group treatment of fibromyalgia: a 6 month outpatient program. J Rheumatol. 1996 Mar;23(3):521–28.

2. Coakley AB, Mahoney EK. Creating a therapeutic and healing environment with a pet therapy program. Complement Ther Clin Pract. 2009 Aug;15(3):141–46.

3. Sim J, Adams N. Physical and other non-pharmacological interventions for fibromyalgia. Baillieres Best Pract Res Clin Rheumatol. 1999 Sep;13(3):507–23.

4. Arnold LM, Clauw DJ, McCarberg BH. Improving the recognition and diagnosis of fibromyalgia. Mayo Clin Proc. 2011 May;86(5):457–64.

5. Pellegrino MJ. Atypical chest pain as an initial presentation of primary fibromyalgia. Arch Phys Med Rehabil. 1990 Jun;71(7):526–28.

6. Peterson EL. Fibromyalgia—management of a misunderstood disorder. J Am Acad Nurse Pract. 2007 Jul;19(7):341–48; Briones-Vozmediano E, Vives-Cases C, Ronda-Pérez E, Gil-González D. Patients' and professionals' views on managing fibromyalgia. Pain Res Manag. 2013 Jan–Feb;18(1):19–24.

7. Hayes SM, Myhal GC, Thornton JF, Camerlain M, Jamison C, Cytryn KN, Murray S. Fibromyalgia and the therapeutic relationship: where uncertainty meets attitude. Pain Res Manag. 2010 Nov–Dec;15(6):385–91.

8. Arnold LM, Clauw DJ, Dunegan LJ, Turk DC; FibroCollaborative. A framework for fibromyalgia management for primary care providers. Mayo Clin Proc. 2012 May;87(5):488–96.

9. Laine C, Turner BJ. The good (gatekeeper), the bad (gatekeeper), and the ugly (situation). J Gen Intern Med. 1999 May;14(5):320–21; Miratashi Yazdi SN, Nedjat S, Arbabi M, Majdzadeh R. Who is a good doctor? Patients & physicians' perspectives. Iran J Public Health. 2015 Jan;44(1):150–52.

10. Beena J, Jose J. Patient medication adherence: measures in daily practice. Oman Med J. 2011 May;26(3):155–59.

11. Offenbächer M, Stucki G. Physical therapy in the treatment of fibromyalgia. Scand J Rheumatol Suppl. 2000;113:78–85; Kaartinen K, Lammi K, Hypen M, Nenonen M, Hanninen O, Rauma AL. Vegan diet alleviates fibromyalgia symptoms. Scand J Rheumatol. 2000;29(5):308–13.

12. Evcik D, Yigit I, Pusak H, Kavuncu V. Effectiveness of aquatic therapy in the treatment of fibromyalgia syndrome: a randomized controlled open study. Rheumatol Int. 2008 Jul;28(9):885–90; Sprott H, Franke S, Kluge H, Hein G. Pain treatment of fibromyalgia by acupuncture. Rheumatol Int. 1998;18(1):35–36.

13. Sim J, Adams N. Therapeutic approaches to fibromyalgia syndrome in the United Kingdom: a survey of occupational therapists and physical therapists. Eur J Pain. 2003;7(2):173–80; Kasper S. The psychiatrist confronted with a fibromyalgia patient. Hum Psychopharmacol. 2009 Jun;24 Suppl 1:S25–30.

14. Arnold LM, Clauw DJ, McCarberg BH; FibroCollaborative. Improving the recognition and diagnosis of fibromyalgia. Mayo Clin Proc. 2011 May;86(5):457–64.

7. ROLES OF FAMILY PHYSICIANS, INTERNISTS, AND NEUROLOGISTS

1. Shleyfer E, Jotkowitz A, Karmon A, Nevzorov R, Cohen H, Buskila D. Accuracy of the diagnosis of fibromyalgia by family physicians: is the pendulum shifting? J Rheumatol. 2009 Jan;36(1):170–73.

2. Jahan F, Nanji K, Qidwai W, Qasim R. Fibromyalgia syndrome: an overview of pathophysiology, diagnosis and management. Oman Med J. 2012 May;27(3):192–95; Evcik D, Kizilay B, Gökçen E. The effects of balneotherapy on fibromyalgia patients. Rheumatol Int. 2002 Jun;22(2):56–59. Epub 2002 Mar 29.

3. Regland B, Andersson M, Abrahamsson L, Bagby J, Dyrehag LE, Gottfries CG. Increased concentrations of homocysteine in the cerebrospinal fluid

in patients with fibromyalgia and Chronic Fatigue Syndrome. Scand J Rheumatol. 1997;26(4):301–7.

4. Eisinger J, Zakarian H, Pouly E, Plantamura A, Ayavou T. Protein peroxidation, magnesium deficiency and fibromyalgia. Magnes Res. 1996 Dec;9(4):313–16.

5. Bellato E, Marini E, Castoldi F, Barbasetti N, Mattei L, Bonasia DE, Blonna D. Fibromyalgia syndrome: etiology, pathogenesis, diagnosis, and treatment. Pain Res Treat. 2012;2012:426130.

6. Hayes SM, Myhal GC, Thornton JF, Camerlain M, Jamison C, Cytryn KN, Murray S. Fibromyalgia and the therapeutic relationship: where uncertainty meets attitude. Pain Res Manag. 2010 Nov–Dec;15(6):385–91.

7. Watson NF, Buchwald D, Goldberg J, Noonan C, Ellenbogen RG. Neurologic signs and symptoms in fibromyalgia. Arthritis Rheum. 2009 Sep;60(9):2839–44.

8. Watson NF, Buchwald D, Goldberg J, Noonan C, Ellenbogen RG. Neurologic signs and symptoms in fibromyalgia. Arthritis Rheum. 2009 Sep;60(9):2839–44.

9. El-Gabalawy H, Ryner L. Central nervous system abnormalities in fibromyalgia: assessment using proton magnetic resonance spectroscopy. J Rheumatol. 2008 Jul;35(7):1242–44; Jahan F, Nanji K, Qidwai W, Qasim R. Fibromyalgia syndrome: an overview of pathophysiology, diagnosis and management. Oman Med J. 2012 May;27(3):192–95.

10. Marcus DA. Fibromyalgia: diagnosis and treatment options. Gend Med. 2009;6 Suppl 2:139–51; Giamberardino MA, Affaitati G, Fabrizio A, Costantini R. Effects of treatment of myofascial trigger points on the pain of fibromyalgia. Curr Pain Headache Rep. 2011 Oct;15(5):393–99; Goldenberg DL. Pharmacological treatment of fibromyalgia and other chronic musculoskeletal pain. Best Pract Res Clin Rheumatol. 2007 Jun;21(3):499–511.

11. Lawson K. Treatment options and patient perspectives in the management of fibromyalgia: future trends. Neuropsychiatr Dis Treat. 2008 Dec;4(6):1059–71.

12. Arnold LM, Clauw DJ, McCarberg BH; FibroCollaborative. Improving the recognition and diagnosis of fibromyalgia. Mayo Clin Proc. 2011 May;86(5):457–64.

13. Clauw DJ. Assessing and diagnosing fibromyalgia in the clinical setting. J Clin Psychiatry. 2008 Nov 6;69(11):e33.

14. Clauw DJ. Assessing and diagnosing fibromyalgia in the clinical setting. J Clin Psychiatry. 2008 Nov 6;69(11):e33.

15. Culpepper L. Recognizing and diagnosing fibromyalgia. J Clin Psychiatry. 2010 Nov;71(11):e30.

8. PREVENTION IS THE KEY

1. Altomonte L, Atzeni F, Leardini G, Marsico A, Gorla R, Casale R, Cassisi G, Stisi S, Salaffi F, Marinangeli F, Giamberardino MA, Di Franco M, Biasi G, Arioli G, Alciati A, Ceccherelli F, Bazzichi L, Carignola R, Cazzola M, Torta R, Buskila D, Spath M, Gracely RH, Sarzi-Puttini P. Fibromyalgia syndrome: preventive, social and economic aspects. Reumatismo. 2008 Jul–Sep;60 Suppl 1:70–78.

2. Sumpton JE, Moulin DE. Fibromyalgia: presentation and management with a focus on pharmacological treatment. Pain Res Manag. 2008 Nov–Dec;13(6):477–83.

3. Vincent A, Benzo RP, Whipple MO, McAllister SJ, Erwin PJ, Saligan LN. Beyond pain in fibromyalgia: insights into the symptom of fatigue. Arthritis Res Ther. 2013;15(6):221.

4. Busch AJ, Webber SC, Brachaniec M, Bidonde J, Bello-Haas VD, Danyliw AD, Overend TJ, Richards RS, Sawant A, Schachter CL. Exercise therapy for fibromyalgia. Curr Pain Headache Rep. 2011 Oct;15(5):358–67; Offenbächer M, Stucki G. Physical therapy in the treatment of fibromyalgia. Scand J Rheumatol Suppl. 2000;113:78–85.

5. Hassett AL, Gevirtz RN. Nonpharmacologic treatment for fibromyalgia: patient education, cognitive-behavioral therapy, relaxation techniques, and complementary and alternative medicine. Rheum Dis Clin North Am. 2009 May;35(2):393–407.

6. Cole RJ. Nonpharmacologic techniques for promoting sleep. Clin Sports Med. 2005 Apr;24(2):343–53, xi.

7. Moldofsky H. Management of sleep disorders in fibromyalgia. Rheum Dis Clin North Am. 2002 May;28(2):353–65.

8. Joseph CL, William LK, Ownby DR, Saltzgaber J, Johnson CC. Applying epidemiologic concepts of primary, secondary, and tertiary prevention to the elimination of racial disparities in asthma. J Allergy Clin Immunol 2006 Feb;117(2):233–40.

9. Vierck CJ. A mechanism-based approach to prevention of and therapy for fibromyalgia. Pain Res Treat. 2012;2012:951354.

10. Thompson RS, Taplin SH, McAfee TA, Mandelson MT, Smith AE. Primary and secondary prevention services in clinical practice. Twenty years' experience in development, implementation, and evaluation. JAMA. 1995 Apr 12;273(14):1130–35.

11. Bondestam E, Hovgren K, Gaston Johansson F, Jern S, Herlitz J, Holmberg S. Pain assessment by patients and nurses in the early phase of acute myocardial infarction. J Adv Nurs. 1987 Nov;12(6):677–82.

12. Dusseldorp E, Klein Velderman M, Paulussen TW, Junger M, van Nieuwenhuijzen M, Reijneveld SA. Targets for primary prevention: cultural, social and intrapersonal factors associated with co-occurring health-related behaviours. Psychol Health. 2014;29(5):598–611.

13. Harth M. Cursing the darkness: reactions to fibromyalgia. Pain Res Manag. 2013 Mar–Apr;18(2):64–66.

14. Bornstein BH, Emler AC, Chapman GB. Rationality in medical treatment decisions: is there a sunk-cost effect? Soc Sci Med. 1999 Jul;49(2):215–22.

15. Age differences in resistance to peer influence.

16. Ogden LL, Richards CL, Shenson D. Clinical preventive services for older adults: the interface between personal health care and public health services. Am J Public Health. 2012 Mar;102(3):419–25.

17. Watson NF, Buchwald D, Goldberg J, Noonan C, Ellenbogen RG. Neurologic signs and symptoms in fibromyalgia. Arthritis Rheum. 2009 Sep;60(9):2839–44.

18. Potter PT, Zautra AJ, Reich JW. Stressful events and information processing dispositions moderate the relationship between positive and negative affect: implications for pain patients. Ann Behav Med. 2000 Summer;22(3):191–98.

19. Spaeth M, Rizzi M, Sarzi-Puttini P. Fibromyalgia and sleep. Best Pract Res Clin Rheumatol. 2011 Apr;25(2):227–39.

20. Chaudhuri A, Behan PO. Fatigue in neurological disorders. Lancet. 2004 Mar 20;363(9413):978–88.

21. Martinez-Lavin M. Biology and therapy of fibromyalgia. Stress, the stress response system, and fibromyalgia. Arthritis Res Ther. 2007;9(4):216.

22. Wahbeh H, Elsas SM, Oken BS. Mind-body interventions: applications in neurology. Neurology. 2008 Jun 10;70(24):2321–28.

23. Choy EH. The role of sleep in pain and fibromyalgia. Nat Rev Rheumatol. 2015 Sept;11(9):513–20.

24. McHugh MP, Magnusson SP, Gleim GW, Nicholas JA. Viscoelastic stress relaxation in human skeletal muscle. Med Sci Sports Exerc. 1992 Dec;24(12):1375–82.

25. Clodomiro A, Gareri P, Puccio G, Frangipane F, Lacava R, Castagna A, Manfredi VG, Colao R, Bruni AC. Somatic comorbidities and Alzheimer's disease treatment. Neurol Sci. 2013 Sep;34(9):1581–89.

26. Letieri RV, Furtado GE, Letieri M, Góes SM, Pinheiro CJ, Veronez SO, Magri AM, Dantas EM. Pain, quality of life, self-perception of health and depression in patients with fibromyalgia, submitted to hydrokinesiotherapy. Rev Bras Reumatol. 2013 Nov–Dec;53(6):494–500.

27. Schmechel DE, Edwards CL. Fibromyalgia, mood disorders, and intense creative energy: A1AT polymorphisms are not always silent. Neurotoxicology. 2012 Dec;33(6):1454–72.

28. Casale R, Rainoldi A. Fatigue and fibromyalgia syndrome: clinical and neurophysiologic pattern. Best Pract Res Clin Rheumatol. 2011 Apr;25(2):241–47.

29. Oechsle K, Wais MC, Vehling S, Bokemeyer C, Mehnert A. Relationship between symptom burden, distress, and sense of dignity in terminally ill cancer patients. J Pain Symptom Manage. 2014 Sep;48(3):313–21.

30. Staines DR. Is fibromyalgia an autoimmune disorder of endogenous vasoactive neuropeptides? Med Hypotheses. 2004;62(5):665–69.

31. Staines DR. Is fibromyalgia an autoimmune disorder of endogenous vasoactive neuropeptides? Med Hypotheses. 2004;62(5):665–69.

9. ALTERNATIVE THERAPIES

1. Tofferi JK, Jackson JL, O'Malley PG. Treatment of fibromyalgia with cyclobenzaprine: A meta-analysis. Arthritis Rheum. 2004 Feb 15;51(1):9–13.

2. Shaver JL, Wilbur J, Lee H, Robinson FP, Wang E. Self-reported medication and herb/supplement use by women with and without fibromyalgia. J Womens Health (Larchmt). 2009 May;18(5):709–16.

3. Dailey DL, Rakel BA, Vance CG, Liebano RE, Amrit AS, Bush HM, Lee KS, Lee JE, Sluka KA. Transcutaneous electrical nerve stimulation reduces pain, fatigue and hyperalgesia while restoring central inhibition in primary fibromyalgia. Pain. 2013 Nov;154(11):2554–62.

4. Staud R. Treatment of fibromyalgia and its symptoms. Expert Opin Pharmacother. 2007 Aug;8(11):1629–42.

5. Casanueva B, Rodero B, Quintial C, Llorca J, González-Gay MA. Short-term efficacy of topical capsaicin therapy in severely affected fibromyalgia patients. Rheumatol Int. 2013 Oct;33(10):2665–70.

6. Chainani-Wu N. Safety and anti-inflammatory activity of curcumin: a component of tumeric (Curcuma longa). J Altern Complement Med. 2003 Feb;9(1):161–68; Chrubasik S. [Devil's claw extract as an example of the effectiveness of herbal analgesics]. Orthopade. 2004 Jul;33(7):804–8; Peloso PM, Khan M, Gross AR, Carlesso L, Santaguida L, Lowcock J, Macdermid JC, Walton D, Goldsmith CH, Langevin P, Shi Q. Pharmacological interventions including medical injections for neck pain: an overview as part of the ICON project. Open Orthop J. 2013 Sep 20;7:473–93.

7. Cabrera C, Artacho R, Giménez R. Beneficial effects of green tea—a review. J Am Coll Nutr. 2006 Apr;25(2):79–99; Srivastava JK, Shankar E, Gup-

ta S. Chamomile: A herbal medicine of the past with bright future. Mol Med Rep. 2010 Nov 1;3(6):895–901; Linde K, Mulrow CD. St John's wort for depression. Cochrane Database Syst Rev. 2000;(2):CD000448.

8. Krenn L. [Passion Flower (Passiflora incarnata L.)—a reliable herbal sedative]. Wien Med Wochenschr. 2002;152(15–16):404–6; Gooneratne NS. Complementary and alternative medicine for sleep disturbances in older adults. Clin Geriatr Med. 2008 Feb;24(1):121–38, viii; Meolie AL, Rosen C, Kristo D, Kohrman M, Gooneratne N, Aguillard RN, Fayle R, Troell R, Townsend D, Claman D, Hoban T, Mahowald M; Clinical Practice Review Committee; American Academy of Sleep Medicine. Oral nonprescription treatment for insomnia: an evaluation of products with limited evidence. J Clin Sleep Med. 2005 Apr 15;1(2):173–87.

9. Li YH, Wang FY, Feng CQ, Yang XF, Sun YH. Massage therapy for fibromyalgia: a systematic review and meta-analysis of randomized controlled trials. PLoS One. 2014 Feb 20;9(2):e89304.

10. Li YH, Wang FY, Feng CQ, Yang XF, Sun YH. Massage therapy for fibromyalgia: a systematic review and meta-analysis of randomized controlled trials. PLoS One. 2014 Feb 20;9(2):e89304.

11. Komarova LA, Zhiganova TI. [Effect of oxygen baths and massage on hemodynamics in patients with neurocirculatory dystonia]. Vopr Kurortol Fizioter Lech Fiz Kult. 2003 Sep–Oct;(5):30–32.

12. Keller G. The effects of massage therapy after decompression and fusion surgery of the lumbar spine: a case study. Int J Ther Massage Bodywork. 2012;5(4):3–8. Epub 2012 Dec 19.

13. Field T, Hernandez-Reif M, Diego M, Schanberg S, Kuhn C. Cortisol decreases and serotonin and dopamine increase following massage therapy. Int J Neurosci. 2005 Oct;115(10):1397–413.

14. Knijnik LM, Dussán-Sarria JA, Rozisky JR, Torres IL, Brunoni AR, Fregni F, Caumo W. Repetitive transcranial magnetic stimulation for fibromyalgia: systematic review and meta-analysis. Pain Pract. 2015 Jan 12.

15. Ernst E. Chiropractic treatment for fibromyalgia: a systematic review. Clin Rheumatol. 2009 Oct;28(10):1175–78.

16. Wong CK. Strain counterstrain: current concepts and clinical evidence. Man Ther. 2012 Feb;17(1):2–8; Day JM, Nitz AJ. The effect of muscle energy techniques on disability and pain scores in individuals with low back pain. J Sport Rehabil. 2012 May;21(2):194–98.

17. Tiidus PM, Shoemaker JK. Effleurage massage, muscle blood flow and long-term post-exercise strength recovery. Int J Sports Med. 1995 Oct;16(7):478–83; Tsao JC. Effectiveness of massage therapy for chronic, non-malignant pain: a review. Evid Based Complement Alternat Med. 2007 Jun;4(2):165–79. Epub 2007 Feb 5; Van Der Riet P. Effleurage and petrissage:

holistic practice in Thailand. Contemp Nurse. 2011 Feb;37(2):227–28; McKechnie GJ, Young WB, Behm DG. Acute effects of two massage techniques on ankle joint flexibility and power of the plantar flexors. J Sports Sci Med. 2007 Dec 1;6(4):498–504. eCollection 2007.

18. Gunnarsdottir TJ, Peden-McAlpine C. Effects of reflexology on fibromyalgia symptoms: a multiple case study. Complement Ther Clin Pract. 2010 Aug;16(3):167–72.

19. Gunnarsdottir TJ, Peden-McAlpine C. Effects of reflexology on fibromyalgia symptoms: a multiple case study. Complement Ther Clin Pract. 2010 Aug;16(3):167–72.

20. Giamberardino MA, Affaitati G, Fabrizio A, Costantini R. Effects of treatment of myofascial trigger points on the pain of fibromyalgia. Curr Pain Headache Rep. 2011 Oct;15(5):393–99.

21. Sprott H, Franke S, Kluge H, Hein G. Pain treatment of fibromyalgia by acupuncture. Rheumatol Int. 1998;18(1):35–36.

22. Chen KW, Hassett AL, Hou F, Staller J, Lichtbroun AS. A pilot study of external qigong therapy for patients with fibromyalgia. J Altern Complement Med. 2006 Nov;12(9):851–56.

23. Jahnke R, Larkey L, Rogers C, Etnier J, Lin F. A comprehensive review of health benefits of qigong and tai chi. Am J Health Promot. 2010 Jul–Aug;24(6):e1–e25.

24. Vincent CA, Richardson PH, Black JJ, Pither CE. The significance of needle placement site in acupuncture. J Psychosom Res. 1989;33(4):489–96.

25. Harris RE, Tian X, Williams DA, Tian TX, Cupps TR, Petzke F, Groner KH, Biswas P, Gracely RH, Clauw DJ. Treatment of fibromyalgia with formula acupuncture: investigation of needle placement, needle stimulation, and treatment frequency. J Altern Complement Med. 2005 Aug;11(4):663–71; Lin D, De La Pena I, Lin L, Zhou SF, Borlongan CV, Cao C. The neuroprotective role of acupuncture and activation of the BDNF signaling pathway. Int J Mol Sci. 2014 Feb 21;15(2):3234–52.

26. Malanga GA, Yan N, Stark J. Mechanisms and efficacy of heat and cold therapies for musculoskeletal injury. Postgrad Med. 2015 Jan;127(1):57–65. Epub 2014 Dec 15.

27. McVeigh JG, McGaughey H, Hall M, Kane P. The effectiveness of hydrotherapy in the management of fibromyalgia syndrome: a systematic review. Rheumatol Int. 2008 Dec;29(2):119–30.

28. Vierck CJ. A mechanism-based approach to prevention of and therapy for fibromyalgia. Pain Res Treat. 2012;2012:951354.

29. Silva A, Queiroz SS, Andersen ML, Mônico-Neto M, Campos RM, Roizenblatt S, Tufik S, Mello MT. Passive body heating improves sleep patterns in female patients with fibromyalgia. Clinics (Sao Paulo). 2013;68(2):135–40.

30. Silva A, Queiroz SS, Andersen ML, Mônico-Neto M, Campos RM, Roizenblatt S, Tufik S, Mello MT. Passive body heating improves sleep patterns in female patients with fibromyalgia. Clinics (Sao Paulo). 2013;68(2):135–40.

31. Offenbächer M, Stucki G. Physical therapy in the treatment of fibromyalgia. Scand J Rheumatol Suppl. 2000;113:78–85.

32. McVeigh JG, McGaughey H, Hall M, Kane P. The effectiveness of hydrotherapy in the management of fibromyalgia syndrome: a systematic review. Rheumatol Int. 2008 Dec;29(2):119–30.

33. Boehm K, Raak C, Cramer H, Lauche R, Ostermann T. Homeopathy in the treatment of fibromyalgia—a comprehensive literature-review and meta-analysis. Complement Ther Med. 2014 Aug;22(4):731–42.

34. Brummett CM, Janda AM, Schueller CM, Tsodikov A, Morris M, Williams DA, Clauw DJ. Survey criteria for fibromyalgia independently predict increased postoperative opioid consumption after lower-extremity joint arthroplasty: a prospective, observational cohort study. Anesthesiology. 2013 Dec;119(6):1434–43.

35. Bellato E, Marini E, Castoldi F, Barbasetti N, Mattei L, Bonasia DE, Blonna D. Fibromyalgia syndrome: etiology, pathogenesis, diagnosis, and treatment. Pain Res Treat. 2012;2012:426130.

36. Cao H, Liu J, Lewith GT. Traditional Chinese Medicine for treatment of fibromyalgia: a systematic review of randomized controlled trials. J Altern Complement Med. 2010 Apr;16(4):397–409; Gooneratne NS. Complementary and alternative medicine for sleep disturbances in older adults. Clin Geriatr Med. 2008 Feb;24(1):121–38, viii.

37. Krenn L. [Passion Flower (Passiflora incarnata L.)—a reliable herbal sedative]. Wien Med Wochenschr. 2002;152(15–16):404–6; Cabrera C, Artacho R, Giménez R. Beneficial effects of green tea—a review. J Am Coll Nutr. 2006 Apr;25(2):79–99; Srivastava JK, Shankar E, Gupta S. Chamomile: A herbal medicine of the past with bright future. Mol Med Rep. 2010 Nov 1;3(6):895–901; Linde K, Mulrow CD, Berner M, Egger, M. St. John's wort for depression. Cochrane Database Syst Rev. 2000 April 18;(2):CD000448.

38. Fernández-San-Martín MI, Masa-Font R, Palacios-Soler L, Sancho-Gómez P, Calbó-Caldentey C, Flores-Mateo G. Effectiveness of Valerian on insomnia: a meta-analysis of randomized placebo-controlled trials. Sleep Med. 2010 Jun;11(6):505–11; Saddichha S. Diagnosis and treatment of chronic insomnia. Ann Indian Acad Neurol. 2010 Apr—Jun;13(2):94–102.

10. CONVENTIONAL TREATMENTS

1. Bellato E, Marini E, Castoldi F, Barbasetti N, Mattei L, Bonasia DE, Blonna D. Fibromyalgia syndrome: etiology, pathogenesis, diagnosis, and treatment. Pain Res Treat. 2012;2012:426130.d.

2. Zimmermann M. Pathophysiological mechanisms of fibromyalgia. Clin J Pain. 1991;7 Suppl 1:S8–15; Maroon JC, Bost JW, Maroon A. Natural anti-inflammatory agents for pain relief. Surg Neurol Int. 2010 Dec 13;1:80; Chandola HC, Chakraborty A. Fibromyalgia and myofascial pain syndrome—a dilemma. Indian J Anaesth. 2009 Oct;53(5):575–81.

3. Hertel J. The role of nonsteroidal anti-inflammatory drugs in the treatment of acute soft tissue injuries. J Athl Train. 1997 Oct;32(4):350–58; Toki M, Aoki K, Katsumi N, Takahashi S. [NSAID and its effect on prostaglandin]. Nihon Rinsho. 2007 Oct;65(10):1807–11.

4. Sumpton JE, Moulin DE. Fibromyalgia: presentation and management with a focus on pharmacological treatment. Pain Res Manag. 2008 Nov–Dec;13(6):477–83; Vaerøy H, Abrahamsen A, Førre O, Kåss E. Treatment of fibromyalgia (fibrositis syndrome): a parallel double blind trial with carisoprodol, paracetamol and caffeine (Somadril comp) versus placebo. Clin Rheumatol. 1989 Jun;8(2):245–50.

5. Argoff CE. Topical analgesics in the management of acute and chronic pain. Mayo Clin Proc. 2013 Feb;88(2):195–205; Needs CJ, Brooks PM. Clinical pharmacokinetics of the salicylates. Clin Pharmacokinet. 1985 Mar–Apr;10(2):164–77; Futami T. [Actions and mechanisms of counterirritants on the muscular circulation]. Nihon Yakurigaku Zasshi. 1984 Mar;83(3):219–26.

6. Guymer EK, Clauw DJ. Treatment of fatigue in fibromyalgia. Rheum Dis Clin North Am. 2002 May;28(2):367–78.

7. Roizenblatt S, Neto NS, Tufik S. Sleep disorders and fibromyalgia. Curr Pain Headache Rep. 2011 Oct;15(5):347–57.

8. Moldofsky H. Management of sleep disorders in fibromyalgia. Rheum Dis Clin North Am. 2002 May;28(2):353–65; Dussias P, Kalali AH, Staud RM. Treatment of fibromyalgia. Psychiatry (Edgmont). 2010 May;7(5):15–18.

9. Rossy LA, Buckelew SP, Dorr N, Hagglund KJ, Thayer JF, McIntosh MJ, Hewett JE, Johnson JC. A meta-analysis of fibromyalgia treatment interventions. Ann Behav Med. 1999 Spring;21(2):180–91.

10. Häuser W, Wolfe F, Tölle T, Uçeyler N, Sommer C. The role of antidepressants in the management of fibromyalgia syndrome: a systematic review and meta-analysis. CNS Drugs. 2012 Apr 1;26(4):297–307; Nishishinya B, Urrútia G, Walitt B, Rodriguez A, Bonfill X, Alegre C, Darko G. Amitriptyline

in the treatment of fibromyalgia: a systematic review of its efficacy. Rheumatology (Oxford). 2008 Dec;47(12):1741–46.

11. Moret C, Briley M. Antidepressants in the treatment of fibromyalgia. Neuropsychiatr Dis Treat. 2006 Dec;2(4):537–48; O'Malley PG, Balden E, Tomkins G, Santoro J, Kroenke K, Jackson JL. Treatment of fibromyalgia with antidepressants: a meta-analysis. J Gen Intern Med. 2000 Sep;15(9):659–66.

12. Lee YC, Chen PP. A review of SSRIs and SNRIs in neuropathic pain. Expert Opin Pharmacother. 2010 Dec;11(17):2813–25.

13. Walitt B, Urrútia G, Nishishinya MB, Cantrell SE, Häuser W. Selective serotonin reuptake inhibitors for fibromyalgia syndrome. Cochrane Database Syst Rev. 2015 Jun 5;6:CD011735.

14. Häuser W, Urrútia G, Tort S, Uçeyler N, Walitt B. Serotonin and noradrenaline reuptake inhibitors (SNRIs) for fibromyalgia syndrome. Cochrane Database Syst Rev. 2013 Jan 31;1:CD010292.

15. Painter JT, Crofford LJ. Chronic opioid use in fibromyalgia syndrome: a clinical review. J Clin Rheumatol. 2013 Mar;19(2):72–77; Üçeyler N, Sommer C, Walitt B, Häuser W. Anticonvulsants for fibromyalgia. Cochrane Database Syst Rev. 2013 Oct 16;10:CD010782.

16. Bennett T, Bray D, Neville MW. Suvorexant, a dual orexin receptor antagonist for the management of insomnia. P T. 2014 Apr;39(4):264–66; Neubauer DN. A review of ramelteon in the treatment of sleep disorders. Neuropsychiatr Dis Treat. 2008 Feb;4(1):69–79; Hajak G, Rodenbeck A, Voderholzer U, Riemann D, Cohrs S, Hohagen F, Berger M, Rüther E. Doxepin in the treatment of primary insomnia: a placebo-controlled, double-blind, polysomnographic study. J Clin Psychiatry. 2001 Jun;62(6):453–63; Roth T, Zorick F, Sicklesteel J, Stepanski E. Effects of benzodiazepines on sleep and wakefulness. Br J Clin Pharmacol. 1981;11 Suppl 1:31S–35S.

17. Richards BL, Whittle SL, Buchbinder R. Muscle relaxants for pain management in rheumatoid arthritis. Cochrane Database Syst Rev. 2012 Jan 18;1:CD008922.

18. [No authors listed]. Understanding fibromyalgia and its related disorders. Prim Care Companion J Clin Psychiatry. 2008;10(2):133–44.

19. Honig PK, Gillespie BK. Drug interactions between prescribed and over-the-counter medication. Drug Saf. 1995 Nov;13(5):296–303; Garcia-Serna R, Mestres J. Anticipating drug side effects by comparative pharmacology. Expert Opin Drug Metab Toxicol. 2010 Oct;6(10):1253–63.

20. Anderson HD, Pace WD, Libby AM, West DR, Valuck RJ. Rates of 5 common antidepressant side effects among new adult and adolescent cases of depression: a retrospective US claims study. Clin Ther. 2012 Jan;34(1):113–23.

21. Makaryus AN, Friedman EA. Patients' understanding of their treatment plans and diagnosis at discharge. Mayo Clin Proc. 2005 Aug;80(8):991–94.

22. Marcus DA. Fibromyalgia: diagnosis and treatment options. Gend Med. 2009;6 Suppl 2:139–51.

23. Goldenberg DL. Pharmacological treatment of fibromyalgia and other chronic musculoskeletal pain. Best Pract Res Clin Rheumatol. 2007 Jun;21(3):499–511.

24. Busch AJ, Webber SC, Brachaniec M, Bidonde J, Bello-Haas VD, Danyliw AD, Overend TJ, Richards RS, Sawant A, Schachter CL. Exercise therapy for fibromyalgia. Curr Pain Headache Rep. 2011 Oct;15(5):358–67.

II. FIBROMYALGIA AND DIET

1. Roberts CK, Barnard RJ. Effects of exercise and diet on chronic disease. J Appl Physiol (1985). 2005 Jan;98(1):3–30.

2. Arranz LI, Canela MA, Rafecas M. Fibromyalgia and nutrition, what do we know? Rheumatol Int. 2010 Sep;30(11):1417–27.

3. Meggs WJ. Neurogenic switching: a hypothesis for a mechanism for shifting the site of inflammation in allergy and chemical sensitivity. Environ Health Perspect. 1995 Jan;103(1):54–56; Sampson HA. Update on food allergy. J Allergy Clin Immunol. 2004 May;113(5):805–19; quiz 820.

4. Staud R. Treatment of fibromyalgia and its symptoms. Expert Opin Pharmacother. 2007 Aug;8(11):1629–42.

5. Cordero MD, de Miguel M, Carmona-López I, Bonal P, Campa F, Moreno-Fernández AM. Oxidative stress and mitochondrial dysfunction in fibromyalgia. Neuro Endocrinol Lett. 2010;31(2):169–73.

6. Hassett AL, Gevirtz RN. Nonpharmacologic treatment for fibromyalgia: patient education, cognitive-behavioral therapy, relaxation techniques, and complementary and alternative medicine. Rheum Dis Clin North Am. 2009 May;35(2):393–407.

7. Donaldson MS, Speight N, Loomis S. Fibromyalgia syndrome improved using a mostly raw vegetarian diet: an observational study. BMC Complement Altern Med. 2001;1:7. Epub 2001 Sep 26; Forman J, Silverstein J; Committee on Nutrition; Council on Environmental Health; American Academy of Pediatrics. Organic foods: health and environmental advantages and disadvantages. Pediatrics. 2012 Nov;130(5):e1406–15; Johnston CS, Steplewska I, Long CA, Harris LN, Ryals RH. Examination of the antiglycemic properties of vinegar in healthy adults. Ann Nutr Metab. 2010;56(1):74–79.

8. Cheuvront SN. The Zone Diet phenomenon: a closer look at the science behind the claims. J Am Coll Nutr. 2003 Feb;22(1):9–17; Austin GL, Ogden LG, Hill JO. Trends in carbohydrate, fat, and protein intakes and association

with energy intake in normal-weight, overweight, and obese individuals: 1971–2006. Am J Clin Nutr. 2011 Apr;93(4):836–43.

9. Christie C. Maintaining a heart-healthy diet most of the time. J Cardiovasc Nurs. 2010 May–Jun;25(3):233–37; Kaartinen K, Lammi K, Hypen M, Nenonen M, Hanninen O, Rauma AL. Vegan diet alleviates fibromyalgia symptoms. Scand J Rheumatol. 2000;29(5):308–13; Willett WC. The Mediterranean diet: science and practice. Public Health Nutr. 2006 Feb;9(1A):105–10; Brand-Miller J, McMillan-Price J, Steinbeck K, Caterson I. Dietary glycemic index: health implications. J Am Coll Nutr. 2009 Aug;28 Suppl:446S–449S.

10. Mengshoel AM, Haugen M. Health status in fibromyalgia—a followup study. J Rheumatol. 2001 Sep;28(9):2085–89.

11. Simopoulos AP. Omega-3 fatty acids in inflammation and autoimmune diseases. J Am Coll Nutr. 2002 Dec;21(6):495–505; Ozgocmen S, Catal SA, Ardicoglu O, Kamanli A. Effect of omega-3 fatty acids in the management of fibromyalgia syndrome. Int J Clin Pharmacol Ther. 2000 Jul;38(7):362–63.

12. Watzl B. Anti-inflammatory effects of plant-based foods and of their constituents. Int J Vitam Nutr Res. 2008 Dec;78(6):293–98; Folchetti LD, Monfort-Pires M, de Barros CR, Martini LA, Ferreira SR. Association of fruits and vegetables consumption and related-vitamins with inflammatory and oxidative stress markers in prediabetic individuals. Diabetol Metab Syndr. 2014 Feb 18;6(1):22.

13. Szatmari SZ, Whitehouse PJ. Vinpocetine for cognitive impairment and dementia Cochrane Database Syst Rev. 2003;(1):CD003119; Ferracioli-Oda E, Qawasmi A, Bloch MH. Meta-analysis: melatonin for the treatment of primary sleep disorders. PLoS One. 2013 May 17;8(5):e63773.

14. Sakarya ST, Akyol Y, Bedir A, Canturk F. The relationship between serum antioxidant vitamins, magnesium levels, and clinical parameters in patients with primary fibromyalgia syndrome. Clin Rheumatol. 2011 Aug;30(8):1039–43.

15. Saha L. Irritable bowel syndrome: pathogenesis, diagnosis, treatment, and evidence-based medicine. World J Gastroenterol. 2014 Jun 14;20(22):6759–73; Kondo M, Hirano Y, Ikai N, Kita K, Jayanegara A, Yokota HO. Assessment of anti-nutritive activity of tannins in tea by-products based on in vitro rumen fermentation. Asian-Australas J Anim Sci. 2014 Nov;27(11):1571–6.

16. Shi Z, Wittert GA, Yuan B, Dai Y, Gill TK, Hu G, Adams R, Zuo H, Taylor AW. Association between monosodium glutamate intake and sleep-disordered breathing among Chinese adults with normal body weight. Nutrition. 2013 Mar;29(3):508–13; Smith JD, Terpening CM, Schmidt SO, Gums JG. Relief of fibromyalgia symptoms following discontinuation of dietary excitotoxins. Ann Pharmacother. 2001 Jun;35(6):702–6; Ciappuccini R, Ansemant

T, Maillefert JF, Tavernier C, Ornetti P. Aspartame-induced fibromyalgia, an unusual but curable cause of chronic pain. Clin Exp Rheumatol. 2010 Nov–Dec;28(6 Suppl 63):S131–3. Epub 2010 Dec 22.

17. Ross AJ, Medow MS, Rowe PC, Stewart JM. What is brain fog? An evaluation of the symptom in postural tachycardia syndrome. Clin Auton Res. 2013 Dec;23(6):305–11.

18. Thornley S, Tayler R, Sikaris K. Sugar restriction: the evidence for a drug-free intervention to reduce cardiovascular disease risk. Intern Med J. 2012 Oct;42 Suppl 5:46–58; White JS. Straight talk about high-fructose corn syrup: what it is and what it ain't. Am J Clin Nutr. 2008 Dec;88(6):1716S–1721S.

19. Albala C, Ebbeling CB, Cifuentes M, Lera L, Bustos N, Ludwig DS. Effects of replacing the habitual consumption of sugar-sweetened beverages with milk in Chilean children. Am J Clin Nutr. 2008 Sep;88(3):605–11; Vartanian LR, Schwartz MB, Brownell KD. Effects of soft drink consumption on nutrition and health: a systematic review and meta-analysis. Am J Public Health. 2007 Apr;97(4):667–75. Epub 2007 Feb 28.

20. Rodrigo L, Blanco I, Bobes J, de Serres FJ. Clinical impact of a gluten-free diet on health-related quality of life in seven fibromyalgia syndrome patients with associated celiac disease. BMC Gastroenterol. 2013 Nov 9;13:157; Ho MH, Wong WH, Chang C. Clinical spectrum of food allergies: a comprehensive review. Clin Rev Allergy Immunol. 2014 Jun;46(3):225–40.

21. Sueiro Blanco F, Estévez Schwarz I, Ayán C, Cancela J, Martín V. Potential benefits of non-pharmacological therapies in fibromyalgia. Open Rheumatol J. 2008;2:1–6.

22. Herman CJ, Allen P, Hunt WC, Prasad A, Brady TJ. Use of complementary therapies among primary care clinic patients with arthritis. Prev Chronic Dis. 2004 Oct;1(4):A12. Epub 2004 Sep 15.

23. Meeusen R. Exercise, nutrition and the brain. Sports Med. 2014 May;44 Suppl 1:S47–56.

24. Massey LK, Whiting SJ. Caffeine, urinary calcium, calcium metabolism and bone. J Nutr. 1993 Sep;123(9):1611–14.

25. Kemper KJ, Shannon S. Complementary and alternative medicine therapies to promote healthy moods. Pediatr Clin North Am. 2007 Dec;54(6):901–26; x; Franco R, Oñatibia-Astibia A, Martínez-Pinilla E. Health benefits of methylxanthines in cacao and chocolate. Nutrients. 2013 Oct 18;5(10):4159–73.

26. Herder R, Demmig-Adams B. The power of a balanced diet and lifestyle in preventing cardiovascular disease. Nutr Clin Care. 2004 Apr–Jun;7(2):46–55; Hu FB, Liu Y, Willett WC. Preventing chronic diseases

by promoting healthy diet and lifestyle: public policy implications for China. Obes Rev. 2011 Jul;12(7):552–59.

27. Sueiro Blanco F, Estévez Schwarz I, Ayán C, Cancela J, Martín V. Potential benefits of non-pharmacological therapies in fibromyalgia. Open Rheumatol J. 2008;2:1–6; Bellato E, Marini E, Castoldi F, Barbasetti N, Mattei L, Bonasia DE, Blonna D. Fibromyalgia syndrome: etiology, pathogenesis, diagnosis, and treatment. Pain Res Treat. 2012;2012:426130.

12. IMPORTANCE OF EXERCISE IN THE TREATMENT OF FM

1. Sharma A, Madaan V, Petty FD. Exercise for mental health. Prim Care Companion J Clin Psychiatry. 2006;8(2):106.

2. Erickson KI, Voss MW, Prakash RS, Basak C, Szabo A, Chaddock L, Kim JS, Heo S, Alves H, White SM, Wojcicki TR, Mailey E, Vieira VJ, Martin SA, Pence BD, Woods JA, McAuley E, Kramer AF. Exercise training increases size of hippocampus and improves memory. Proc Natl Acad Sci U S A. 2011 Feb 15;108(7):3017–22.

3. Penedo FJ, Dahn JR. Exercise and well-being: a review of mental and physical health benefits associated with physical activity. Curr Opin Psychiatry. 2005 Mar;18(2):189–93; Mischel NA, Llewellyn-Smith IJ, Mueller PJ. Physical (in)activity-dependent structural plasticity in bulbospinal catecholaminergic neurons of rat rostral ventrolateral medulla. J Comp Neurol. 2014 Feb 15;522(3):499–513.

4. Agudelo LZ, Femenía T, Orhan F, Porsmyr-Palmertz M, Goiny M, Martinez-Redondo V, Correia JC, Izadi M, Bhat M, Schuppe-Koistinen I, Pettersson AT, Ferreira DM, Krook A, Barres R, Zierath JR, Erhardt S, Lindskog M, Ruas JL. Skeletal muscle PGC-1α1 modulates kynurenine metabolism and mediates resilience to stress-induced depression. Cell. 2014 Sep 25;159(1):33–45.

5. Dobson JL, McMillan J, Li L. Benefits of exercise intervention in reducing neuropathic pain. Front Cell Neurosci. 2014 Apr 4;8:102.

6. Offenbächer M, Stucki G. Physical therapy in the treatment of fibromyalgia. Scand J Rheumatol Suppl. 2000;113:78–85.

7. Giannotti E, Koutsikos K, Pigatto M, Rampudda ME, Doria A, Masiero S. Medium-/long-term effects of a specific exercise protocol combined with patient education on spine mobility, chronic fatigue, pain, aerobic fitness and level of disability in fibromyalgia. Biomed Res Int. 2014;2014:474029.

8. Yaffe K, Barnes D, Nevitt M, Lui LY, Covinsky K. A prospective study of physical activity and cognitive decline in elderly women: women who walk. Arch Intern Med. 2001 Jul 23;161(14):1703–8; Dimeo F, Bauer M, Varahram

I, Proest G, Halter U. Benefits from aerobic exercise in patients with major depression: a pilot study. Br J Sports Med. 2001 Apr;35(2):114–17; Meyer BB, Lemley KJ. Utilizing exercise to affect the symptomology of fibromyalgia: a pilot study. Med Sci Sports Exerc. 2000 Oct;32(10):1691–97.

9. Carson JW, Carson KM, Jones KD, Bennett RM, Wright CL, Mist SD. A pilot randomized controlled trial of the Yoga of Awareness program in the management of fibromyalgia. Pain. 2010 Nov;151(2):530–39; Pekmezi D, Martin MY, Kvale E, Meneses K, Demark-Wahnefried W. Enhancing exercise adherence for the breast cancer survivors. ACSMs Health Fit J. 2012 Jul 1;16(4):8–13; Staples JK, Hamilton MF, Uddo M. A yoga program for the symptoms of post-traumatic stress disorder in veterans. Mil Med. 2013 Aug;178(8):854–60.

10. Evcik D, Yigit I, Pusak H, Kavuncu V. Effectiveness of aquatic therapy in the treatment of fibromyalgia syndrome: a randomized controlled open study. Rheumatol Int. 2008 Jul;28(9):885–90; Tomas-Carus P, Gusi N, Häkkinen A, Häkkinen K, Leal A, Ortega-Alonso A. Eight months of physical training in warm water improves physical and mental health in women with fibromyalgia: a randomized controlled trial. J Rehabil Med. 2008 Apr;40(4):248–52.

11. Buettner LL, Fitzsimmons S. AD-venture program: therapeutic biking for the treatment of depression in long-term care residents with dementia. Am J Alzheimers Dis Other Demen. 2002 Mar–Apr;17(2):121–27; Erickson KI, Prakash RS, Voss MW, Chaddock L, Hu L, Morris KS, White SM, Wójcicki TR, McAuley E, Kramer AF. Aerobic fitness is associated with hippocampal volume in elderly humans. Hippocampus. 2009 Oct;19(10):1030–39.

12. Altan L, Korkmaz N, Bingol U, Gunay B. Effect of pilates training on people with fibromyalgia syndrome: a pilot study. Arch Phys Med Rehabil. 2009 Dec;90(12):1983–88.

13. Daenen L, Varkey E, Kellmann M, Nijs J. Exercise, not to exercise, or how to exercise in patients with chronic pain? Applying science to practice. Clin J Pain. 2015 Feb;31(2):108–14.

14. Jones KD. Nordic walking in fibromyalgia: a means of promoting fitness that is easy for busy clinicians to recommend. Arthritis Res Ther. 2011 Feb 16;13(1):103.

15. Binder AI. Cervical spondylosis and neck pain. BMJ. 2007 Mar 10;334(7592):527–31.

16. Busch AJ, Webber SC, Brachaniec M, Bidonde J, Bello-Haas VD, Danyliw AD, Overend TJ, Richards RS, Sawant A, Schachter CL. Exercise therapy for fibromyalgia. Curr Pain Headache Rep. 2011 Oct;15(5):358–67.

17. Baptista AS, Villela AL, Jones A, Natour J. Effectiveness of dance in patients with fibromyalgia: a randomized, single-blind, controlled study. Clin Exp Rheumatol. 2012 Nov–Dec;30(6 Suppl 74):18–23. Epub 2012 Dec 14.

18. Jones KD, Liptan GL. Exercise interventions in fibromyalgia: clinical applications from the evidence. Rheum Dis Clin North Am. 2009 May;35(2):373–91; Häuser W, Klose P, Langhorst J, Moradi B, Steinbach M, Schiltenwolf M, Busch A. Efficacy of different types of aerobic exercise in fibromyalgia syndrome: a systematic review and meta-analysis of randomised controlled trials. Arthritis Res Ther. 2010;12(3):R79.

19. Ross RL, Jones KD, Bennett RM, Ward RL, Druker BJ, Wood LJ. Preliminary evidence of increased pain and elevated cytokines in fibromyalgia patients with defective growth hormone response to exercise. Open Immunol J. 2010;3:9–18.Brooks K, Carter J. Overtraining, Exercise, and Adrenal Insufficiency. J Nov Physiother. 2013 Feb 16;3(125);ii: 11717.

20. Martin L, Nutting A, MacIntosh BR, Edworthy SM, Butterwick D, Cook J. An exercise program in the treatment of fibromyalgia. J Rheumatol. 1996 Jun;23(6):1050–53.

13. LENDING A HELPING HAND

1. Khamis V. Post-traumatic stress disorder among school age Palestinian children. Child Abuse Negl. 2005 Jan;29(1):81–95; Kurtze N, Gundersen KT, Svebak S. Quality of life, functional disability and lifestyle among subgroups of fibromyalgia patients: the significance of anxiety and depression. Br J Med Psychol. 1999 Dec;72 (Pt 4):471–84.

2. [No authors listed]. Understanding fibromyalgia and its related disorders. Prim Care Companion J Clin Psychiatry. 2008;10(2):133–44; Hallberg LR, Carlsson SG. Coping with fibromyalgia. A qualitative study. Scand J Caring Sci. 2000;14(1):29–36.

3. Henriksson C, Gundmark I, Bengtsson A, Ek AC. Living with fibromyalgia. Consequences for everyday life. Clin J Pain. 1992 Jun;8(2):138–44.

4. Van Uden-Kraan CF, Drossaert CH, Taal E, Shaw BR, Seydel ER, van de Laar MA. Empowering processes and outcomes of participation in online support groups for patients with breast cancer, arthritis, or fibromyalgia. Qual Health Res. 2008 Mar;18(3):405–17.

5. Friedberg F, Leung DW, Quick J. Do support groups help people with chronic fatigue syndrome and fibromyalgia? A comparison of active and inactive members. J Rheumatol. 2005 Dec;32(12):2416–20; van Uden-Kraan CF, Drossaert CH, Taal E, Shaw BR, Seydel ER, van de Laar MA. Empowering processes and outcomes of participation in online support groups for patients

with breast cancer, arthritis, or fibromyalgia. Qual Health Res. 2008 Mar;18(3):405–17.

6. Annemans L, Le Lay K, Taïeb C. Societal and patient burden of fibromyalgia syndrome. Pharmacoeconomics. 2009;27(7):547–59.

7. Friedberg F, Leung DW, Quick J. Do support groups help people with chronic fatigue syndrome and fibromyalgia? A comparison of active and inactive members. J Rheumatol. 2005 Dec;32(12):2416–20; van Uden-Kraan CF, Drossaert CH, Taal E, Shaw BR, Seydel ER, van de Laar MA. Empowering processes and outcomes of participation in online support groups for patients with breast cancer, arthritis, or fibromyalgia. Qual Health Res. 2008 Mar;18(3):405–17.

8. Fitzcharles MA, Shir Y, Ablin JN, Buskila D, Amital H, Henningsen P, Häuser W. Classification and clinical diagnosis of fibromyalgia syndrome: recommendations of recent evidence-based interdisciplinary guidelines. Evid Based Complement Alternat Med. 2013;2013:528952; Wolfe F, Walitt BT, Katz RS, Häuser W. Symptoms, the nature of fibromyalgia, and *Diagnostic and Statistical Manual* 5 (DSM-5) defined mental illness in patients with rheumatoid arthritis and fibromyalgia. PLoS One. 2014 Feb 14;9(2):e88740.

9. James C, MacKenzie L. The clinical utility of functional capacity evaluations: the opinion of health professionals working within occupational rehabilitation. Work. 2009;33(3):231–39.

10. Lavergne MR, Cole DC, Kerr K, Marshall LM. Functional impairment in chronic fatigue syndrome, fibromyalgia, and multiple chemical sensitivity. Can Fam Physician. 2010 Feb;56(2):e57–65.

11. Rashid A. Finance, fibromyalgia, caring, & communication. Br J Gen Pract. 2014 May;64(622):244.

12. Briones-Vozmediano E, Vives-Cases C, Ronda-Pérez E, Gil-González D. Patients' and professionals' views on managing fibromyalgia. Pain Res Manag. 2013 Jan–Feb;18(1):19–24.

13. Clauw DJ, Arnold LM, McCarberg BH; FibroCollaborative. The science of fibromyalgia. Mayo Clin Proc. 2011 Sep;86(9):907–11.

14. APPROACHING THE MENTAL ASPECTS

1. Okifuji A, Turk DC, Sherman JJ. Evaluation of the relationship between depression and fibromyalgia syndrome: why aren't all patients depressed? J Rheumatol. 2000 Jan;27(1):212–19.

2. Goldberg S. Talk therapy vs drug therapy for depression. Arch Gen Psychiatry. 1987 Oct;44(10):923.

3. Fava GA, Rafanelli C, Grandi S, Conti S, Belluardo P. Prevention of recurrent depression with cognitive behavioral therapy: preliminary findings. Arch Gen Psychiatry. 1998 Sep;55(9):816–20.

4. Markowitz JC, Weissman MM. Interpersonal psychotherapy: principles and applications. World Psychiatry. 2004 Oct;3(3):136–39.

5. Ali BS, Rahbar MH, Naeem S, Gul A, Mubeen S, Iqbal A. The effectiveness of counseling on anxiety and depression by minimally trained counselors: a randomized controlled trial. Am J Psychother. 2003;57(3):324–36.

6. Ferguson JM. SSRI antidepressant medications: adverse effects and tolerability. Prim Care Companion J Clin Psychiatry. 2001 Feb;3(1):22–27.

7. Hirschfeld RM. Efficacy of SSRIs and newer antidepressants in severe depression: comparison with TCAs. J Clin Psychiatry. 1999 May;60(5):326–35.

8. Schug SA. The role of tramadol in current treatment strategies for musculoskeletal pain. Ther Clin Risk Manag. 2007 Oct;3(5):717–23.

9. Segura-Jiménez V, Camiletti-Moirón D, Munguía-Izquierdo D, Álvarez-Gallardo IC, Ruiz JR, Ortega FB, Delgado-Fernández M. Agreement between self-reported sleep patterns and actigraphy in fibromyalgia and healthy women. Clin Exp Rheumatol. 2015 Jan–Feb;33(1 Suppl 88):S58–67. Epub 2015 Mar 18.

10. Ang DC, Kaleth AS, Bigatti S, Mazzuca SA, Jensen MP, Hilligoss J, Slaven J, Saha C. Research to encourage exercise for fibromyalgia (REEF): use of motivational interviewing, outcomes from a randomized-controlled trial. Gen Hosp Psychiatry. 2013 Apr;29(4):296–304.

11. Jorm AF, Griffiths KM, Christensen H, Parslow RA, Rogers B. Actions taken to cope with depression at different levels of severity: a community survey. Psychol Med. 2004 Feb;34(2):293–99; Dirmaier J, Steinmann M, Krattenmacher T, Watzke B, Barghaan D, Koch U, Schulz H. Non-pharmacological treatment of depressive disorders: a review of evidence-based treatment options. Rev Recent Clin Trials. 2012 May;7(2):141–49.

12. Mahdi AA, Fatima G, Das SK, Verma NS. Abnormality of circadian rhythm of serum melatonin and other biochemical parameters in fibromyalgia syndrome. Indian J Biochem Biophys. 2011 Apr;48(2):82–87.

13. Miklowitz DJ, Price J, Holmes EA, Rendell J, Bell S, Budge K, Christensen J, Wallace J, Simon J, Armstrong NM, McPeake L, Goodwin GM, Geddes JR. Facilitated Integrated Mood Management for adults with bipolar disorder. Bipolar Disord. 2012 Mar;14(2):185–97; Benton D. Carbohydrate ingestion, blood glucose and mood. Neurosci Biobehav Rev. 2002 May;26(3):293–308.

14. Smith RA, Lack LC, Lovato N, Wright H. The relationship between a night's sleep and subsequent daytime functioning in older poor and good sleepers. J Sleep Res. 2015 Feb;24(1):40–46.

15. Otto MW, Church TS, Craft LL, Greer TL, Smits JA, Trivedi MH. Exercise for mood and anxiety disorders. Prim Care Companion J Clin Psychiatry. 2007;9(4):287–94.

16. Murrock CJ, Higgins PA. The theory of music, mood and movement to improve health outcomes. J Adv Nurs. 2009 Oct;65(10):2249–57.

17. Casini ML, Marelli G, Papaleo E, Ferrari A, D'Ambrosio F, Unfer V. Psychological assessment of the effects of treatment with phytoestrogens on postmenopausal women: a randomized, double-blind, crossover, placebo-controlled study. Fertil Steril. 2006 Apr;85(4):972–8.

18. Linde K, Mulrow CD. St John's wort for depression. Cochrane Database Syst Rev. 2000;(2):CD000448.

19. Casale R, Cazzola M, Arioli G, Gracely RH, Ceccherelli F, Atzeni F, Stisi S, Cassisi G, Altomonte L, Alciati A, Leardini G, Gorla R, Marsico A, Torta R, Giamberardino MA, Buskila D, Spath M, Marinangeli F, Bazzichi L, Di Franco M, Biasi G, Salaffi F, Carignola R, Sarzi-Puttini P; Italian Fibromyalgia Network. Non pharmacological treatments in fibromyalgia. Reumatismo. 2008 Jul–Sep;60 Suppl 1:59–69.

20. Ariga A, Lleras A. Brief and rare mental "breaks" keep you focused: deactivation and reactivation of task goals preempt vigilance decrements. Cognition. 2011 Mar;118(3):439–43.

21. Sharma A, Madaan V, Petty FD. Exercise for mental health. Prim Care Companion J Clin Psychiatry. 2006;8(2):106.

22. Gómez-Pinilla F. Brain foods: the effects of nutrients on brain function. Nat Rev Neurosci. 2008 Jul;9(7):568–78.

23. Sharma A, Madaan V, Petty FD. Exercise for mental health. Prim Care Companion J Clin Psychiatry. 2006;8(2):106.

24. Lumley MA. Beyond cognitive-behavioral therapy for fibromyalgia: addressing stress by emotional exposure, processing, and resolution. Arthritis Res Ther. 2011;13(6):136; Ko HJ, Youn CH. Effects of laughter therapy on depression, cognition and sleep among the community-dwelling elderly. Geriatr Gerontol Int. 2011 Jul;11(3):267–74.

25. Jäncke L. Music, memory and emotion. J Biol. 2008 Aug 8;7(6):21.

26. Sharma NK, Robbins K, Wagner K, Colgrove YM. A randomized controlled pilot study of the therapeutic effects of yoga in people with Parkinson's disease. Int J Yoga. 2015 Jan;8(1):74–79;Gunther KL. The use of "non-fiction novels" in a sensation and perception course. J Undergrad Neurosci Educ. 2011 Oct 15;10(1):A14–23. Print 2011 Fall.

27. Parra A. A common role for psychotropic medications: memory impairment. Med Hypotheses. 2003 Jan;60(1):133–42.

28. Arnold LM. Strategies for managing fibromyalgia. Am J Med. 2009 Dec;122(12 Suppl):S31–43.

15. BEING A PARENT WITH FIBROMYALGIA

1. Sil S, Lynch-Jordan A, Ting TV, Peugh J, Noll J, Kashikar-Zuck S. Influence of family environment on long-term psychosocial functioning of adolescents with juvenile fibromyalgia. Arthritis Care Res (Hoboken). 2013 Jun;65(6):903–9.

2. Kool MB, van Middendorp H, Boeije HR, Geenen R. Understanding the lack of understanding: invalidation from the perspective of the patient with fibromyalgia. Arthritis Rheum. 2009 Dec 15;61(12):1650–56.

3. Hallberg LR, Carlsson SG. Coping with fibromyalgia. A qualitative study. Scand J Caring Sci. 2000;14(1):29–36.

4. Reid GJ, McGrath PJ, Lang BA. Parent-child interactions among children with juvenile fibromyalgia, arthritis, and healthy controls. Pain. 2005 Jan;113(1–2):201–10.

5. Smith M. Good parenting: Making a difference. Early Hum Dev. 2010 Nov;86(11):689–93.

6. Henwood K, Procter J. The "good father": reading men's accounts of paternal involvement during the transition to first-time fatherhood. Br J Soc Psychol. 2003 Sep;42(Pt 3):337–55.

7. Welles-Nyström B, New R, Richman A. The "good mother"—a comparative study of Swedish, Italian and American maternal behavior and goals. Scand J Caring Sci. 1994;8(2):81–86; Poduval J, Poduval M. Working mothers: how much working, how much mothers, and where is the womanhood? Mens Sana Monogr. 2009 Jan–Dec;7(1):63–79.

8. Collado A, Gomez E, Coscolla R, Sunyol R, Solé E, Rivera J, Altarriba E, Carbonell J, Castells X. Work, family and social environment in patients with fibromyalgia in Spain: an epidemiological study: EPIFFAC study. BMC Health Serv Res. 2014 Nov 11;14:513; Lewis FM, Woods NF, Hough EE, Bensley LS. The family's functioning with chronic illness in the mother: the spouse's perspective. Soc Sci Med. 1989;29(11):1261–69.

9. Freer CB. Health diaries: a method of collecting health information. J R Coll Gen Pract. 1980 May;30(214):279–82.

10. Collado A, Gomez E, Coscolla R, Sunyol R, Solé E, Rivera J, Altarriba E, Carbonell J, Castells X. Work, family and social environment in patients with fibromyalgia in Spain: an epidemiological study: EPIFFAC study. BMC Health Serv Res. 2014 Nov 11;14:513; Häuser W, Arnold B, Eich W, Felde E, Flügge C, Henningsen P, Herrmann M, Köllner V, Kühn E, Nutzinger D, Offenbächer M, Schiltenwolf M, Sommer C, Thieme K, Kopp I. Management of fibromyalgia syndrome—an interdisciplinary evidence-based guideline. Ger Med Sci. 2008 Dec 9;6:Doc14.

11. Häuser W, Eich W, Herrmann M, Nutzinger DO, Schiltenwolf M, Henningsen P. Fibromyalgia syndrome: classification, diagnosis, and treatment. Dtsch Arztebl Int. 2009 Jun;106(23):383–91.

12. Schaefer KM. Breastfeeding in chronic illness: the voices of women with fibromyalgia. MCN Am J Matern Child Nurs. 2004 Jul–Aug;29(4):248–53.

13. Datler W, Ereky-Stevens K, Hover-Reisner N, Malmberg LE. Toddlers' transition to out-of-home day care: settling into a new care environment. Infant Behav Dev. 2012 Jun;35(3):439–51.

14. Kieckhefer GM, Trahms CM, Churchill SS, Simpson JN. Measuring parent-child shared management of chronic illness. Pediatr Nurs. 2009 Mar–Apr;35(2):101–8, 127.

15. DeVore ER, Ginsburg KR. The protective effects of good parenting on adolescents. Curr Opin Pediatr. 2005 Aug;17(4):460–65.

16. FIBROMYALGIA-RELATED OCCUPATIONAL CONSTRAINTS

1. Bernard AL, Prince A, Edsall P. Quality of life issues for fibromyalgia patients. Arthritis Care Res. 2000 Feb;13(1):42–50; Jäckel WH, Genth E. [Fibromyalgia]. Z Rheumatol. 2007 Nov;66(7):579–90.

2. Mannerkorpi K, Gard G. Hinders for continued work among persons with fibromyalgia. BMC Musculoskelet Disord. 2012 Jun 11;13:96.

3. Glass JM. Fibromyalgia and cognition. J Clin Psychiatry. 2008;69 Suppl 2:20–24; Seo J, Kim SH, Kim YT, Song HJ, Lee JJ, Kim SH, Han SW, Nam EJ, Kim SK, Lee HJ, Lee SJ, Chang Y. Working memory impairment in fibromyalgia patients associated with altered frontoparietal memory network. PLoS One. 2012;7(6):e37808.

4. Chandran A, Schaefer C, Ryan K, Baik R, McNett M, Zlateva G. The comparative economic burden of mild, moderate, and severe fibromyalgia: results from a retrospective chart review and cross-sectional survey of working-age U.S. adults. J Manag Care Pharm. 2012 Jul–Aug;18(6):415–26.

5. Skaer TL. Fibromyalgia: disease synopsis, medication cost effectiveness and economic burden. Pharmacoeconomics. 2014 May;32(5):457–66; Perrot S, Schaefer C, Knight T, Hufstader M, Chandran AB, Zlateva G. Societal and individual burden of illness among fibromyalgia patients in France: association between disease severity and OMERACT core domains. BMC Musculoskelet Disord. 2012 Feb 17;13:22.

6. [No authors listed]. Understanding fibromyalgia and its related disorders. Prim Care Companion J Clin Psychiatry. 2008;10(2):133–44; de Vries HJ, Reneman MF, Groothoff JW, Geertzen JH, Brouwer S. Self-reported work

ability and work performance in workers with chronic nonspecific musculoskeletal pain. J Occup Rehabil. 2013 Mar;23(1):1–10.

7. Michielsen HJ, Van Houdenhove B, Leirs I, Vandenbroeck A, Onghena P. Depression, attribution style and self-esteem in chronic fatigue syndrome and fibromyalgia patients: is there a link? Clin Rheumatol. 2006 Mar;25(2):183–8.

8. Martinez-Lavin M. Fibromyalgia: when distress becomes (un)sympathetic pain. Pain Res Treat. 2012;2012:981565; Kivimäki M, Leino-Arjas P, Kaila-Kangas L, Virtanen M, Elovainio M, Puttonen S, Keltikangas-Järvinen L, Pentti J, Vahtera J. Increased absence due to sickness among employees with fibromyalgia. Ann Rheum Dis. 2007 Jan;66(1):65–9. Epub 2006 Jun 22.

9. Castro-Sánchez AM, Matarán-Peñarrocha GA, Granero-Molina J, Aguilera-Manrique G, Quesada-Rubio JM, Moreno-Lorenzo C. Benefits of massage-myofascial release therapy on pain, anxiety, quality of sleep, depression, and quality of life in patients with fibromyalgia. Evid Based Complement Alternat Med. 2011;2011:561753.

10. Briones-Vozmediano E, Ronda-Pérez E, Vives-Cases C. [Fibromyalgia patients' perceptions of the impact of the disease in the workplace]. Aten Primaria. 2015 Apr;47(4):205–12; Kivimäki M, Leino-Arjas P, Virtanen M, Elovainio M, Keltikangas-Järvinen L, Puttonen S, Vartia M, Brunner E, Vahtera J. Work stress and incidence of newly diagnosed fibromyalgia: prospective cohort study. J Psychosom Res. 2004 Nov;57(5):417–22.

11. Munyewende PO, Rispel LC. Using diaries to explore the work experiences of primary health care nursing managers in two South African provinces. Glob Health Action. 2014 Dec 22;7:25323.

12. Löfgren M, Ekholm J, Ohman A. "A constant struggle": successful strategies of women in work despite fibromyalgia. Disabil Rehabil. 2006 Apr 15;28(7):447–55.

13. da Costa BR, Vieira ER. Stretching to reduce work-related musculoskeletal disorders: a systematic review. J Rehabil Med. 2008 May;40(5):321–28; Merrill RM, Aldana SG, Garrett J, Ross C. Effectiveness of a workplace wellness program for maintaining health and promoting healthy behaviors. J Occup Environ Med. 2011 Jul;53(7):782–87.

14. Hassett AL, Gevirtz RN. Nonpharmacologic treatment for fibromyalgia: patient education, cognitive-behavioral therapy, relaxation techniques, and complementary and alternative medicine. Rheum Dis Clin North Am. 2009 May;35(2):393–407; Bohay M, Blakely DP, Tamplin AK, Radvansky GA. Note taking, review, memory, and comprehension. Am J Psychol. 2011 Spring;124(1):63–73.

15. Reilly PA . Fibromyalgia in the workplace: a "management" problem. Ann Rheum Dis. 1993 Apr;52(4):249–51; Mannerkorpi K, Ekdahl C. Assessment of functional limitation and disability in patients with fibromyalgia. Scand J Rheumatol. 1997;26(1):4–13.

17. CONCLUSION

1. Beal CC, Stuifbergen AK, Brown A. Predictors of a health promoting lifestyle in women with fibromyalgia syndrome. Psychol Health Med. 2009 May;14(3):343–53.

2. Mishra SK, Singh P, Bunch SJ, Zhang R. The therapeutic value of yoga in neurological disorders. Ann Indian Acad Neurol. 2012 Oct;15(4):247–54.

3. Theadom A, Cropley M, Kantermann T. Daytime napping associated with increased symptom severity in fibromyalgia syndrome. BMC Musculoskelet Disord. 2015 Feb 7;16:13.

4. Orlandi AC, Ventura C, Gallinaro AL, Costa RA, Lage LV. Improvement in pain, fatigue, and subjective sleep quality through sleep hygiene tips in patients with fibromyalgia. Rev Bras Reumatol. 2012 Oct;52(5):666–78; Li YH, Wang FY, Feng CQ, Yang XF, Sun YH. Massage therapy for fibromyalgia: a systematic review and meta-analysis of randomized controlled trials. PLoS One. 2014 Feb 20;9(2):e89304.

5. Vaerøy H, Abrahamsen A, Førre O, Kåss E. Treatment of fibromyalgia (fibrositis syndrome): a parallel double blind trial with carisoprodol, paracetamol and caffeine (Somadril comp) versus placebo. Clin Rheumatol. 1989 Jun;8(2):245–50; Holton KF, Taren DL, Thomson CA, Bennett RM, Jones KD. The effect of dietary glutamate on fibromyalgia and irritable bowel symptoms. Clin Exp Rheumatol. 2012 Nov–Dec;30(6 Suppl 74):10–17.

6. Friedberg F, Williams DA, Collinge W. Lifestyle-oriented non-pharmacological treatments for fibromyalgia: a clinical overview and applications with home-based technologies. J Pain Res. 2012;5:425–35.

7. Rau J, Ehlebracht-König I, Petermann F. [Impact of a motivational intervention on coping with chronic pain: results of a controlled efficacy study]. Schmerz. 2008 Oct;22(5):575–78, 580–85.

8. Rau J, Ehlebracht-König I, Petermann F. [Impact of a motivational intervention on coping with chronic pain: results of a controlled efficacy study]. Schmerz. 2008 Oct;22(5):575–78, 580–85.

9. van Middendorp H, Lumley MA, Jacobs JW, van Doornen LJ, Bijlsma JW, Geenen R. Emotions and emotional approach and avoidance strategies in fibromyalgia. J Psychosom Res. 2008 Feb;64(2):159–67.

10. Hammond A, Freeman K. Community patient education and exercise for people with fibromyalgia: a parallel group randomized controlled trial. Clin Rehabil. 2006 Oct;20(10):835–46.

11. Pastor MÁ, López-Roig S, Lledó A, Peñacoba C, Velasco L, Schweiger-Gallo I, Cigarán M, Ecija C, Limón R, Sanz Y. Combining motivational and volitional strategies to promote unsupervised walking in patients with fibromyalgia: study protocol for a randomized controlled trial. Trials. 2014 Apr 11;15:120.

12. Thieme K, Turk DC, Gracely RH, Maixner W, Flor H. The relationship among psychological and psychophysiological characteristics of fibromyalgia patients. J Pain. 2015 Feb;16(2):186–96.

13. Swisher AK. Patience and patients. Cardiopulm Phys Ther J. 2013 Jun;24(2):4.

14. Seo J, Kim SH, Kim YT, Song HJ, Lee JJ, Kim SH, Han SW, Nam EJ, Kim SK, Lee HJ, Lee SJ, Chang Y. Working memory impairment in fibromyalgia patients associated with altered frontoparietal memory network. PLoS One. 2012;7(6):e37808.

15. White LA, Birnbaum HG, Kaltenboeck A, Tang J, Mallett D, Robinson RL. Employees with fibromyalgia: medical comorbidity, healthcare costs, and work loss. J Occup Environ Med. 2008 Jan;50(1):13–24.

16. Carson AJ, Ringbauer B, MacKenzie L, Warlow C, Sharpe M. Neurological disease, emotional disorder, and disability: they are related: a study of 300 consecutive new referrals to a neurology outpatient department. J Neurol Neurosurg Psychiatry. 2000 Feb;68(2):202–6.

17. Sicras-Mainar A, Rejas J, Navarro R, Blanca M, Morcillo A, Larios R, Velasco S, Villarroya C. Treating patients with fibromyalgia in primary care settings under routine medical practice: a claim database cost and burden of illness study. Arthritis Res Ther. 2009;11(2):R54.

18. Vowles KE, McCracken LM, Eccleston C. Patient functioning and catastrophizing in chronic pain: the mediating effects of acceptance. Health Psychol. 2008 Mar;27(2 Suppl):S136–43.

19. Häuser W, Arnold B, Eich W, Felde E, Flügge C, Henningsen P, Herrmann M, Köllner V, Kühn E, Nutzinger D, Offenbächer M, Schiltenwolf M, Sommer C, Thieme K, Kopp I. Management of fibromyalgia syndrome—an interdisciplinary evidence-based guideline. Ger Med Sci. 2008 Dec 9;6:Doc14.

20. Sicras-Mainar A, Rejas J, Navarro R, Blanca M, Morcillo A, Larios R, Velasco S, Villarroya C. Treating patients with fibromyalgia in primary care settings under routine medical practice: a claim database cost and burden of illness study. Arthritis Res Ther. 2009;11(2):R54.

21. Ha JF, Longnecker N. Doctor-patient communication: a review. Ochsner J. 2010 Spring;10(1):38–43.

22. Briones-Vozmediano E, Vives-Cases C, Ronda-Pérez E, Gil-González D. Patients' and professionals' views on managing fibromyalgia. Pain Res Manag. 2013 Jan–Feb;18(1):19–24.

23. Lantelme P, Milon H, Gharib C, Gayet C, Fortrat JO. White coat effect and reactivity to stress: cardiovascular and autonomic nervous system responses. Hypertension. 1998 Apr;31(4):1021–29.

24. Fontaine KR, Conn L, Clauw DJ. Effects of lifestyle physical activity in adults with fibromyalgia: results at follow-up. J Clin Rheumatol. 2011 Mar;17(2):64–68.

GLOSSARY OF TERMS

Abscess—a localized collection of pus on the skin that generally occurs due to an infection.

Acute—a short-lasting, rapid onset of a disease.

Adrenaline—a hormone that stimulates the sympathetic nervous system to increase heart rate, blood flow, and energy stores in the body. Adrenaline is released in response to stressful situations, such as those relating to the survival "fight-or-flight" phenomenon.

Allodynia—pain from a stimulus that is not normally painful.

Alzheimer's—a disease that accompanies mental confusion and memory loss. This is a disease that progressively gets worse with age.

Analgesics—drugs used for pain relief.

Angina—chest pain resulting from a lack of oxygen-rich blood flowing to the heart.

Apoplexy—a loss in neurological function generally due to lack of blood flow to the brain (i.e., stroke, brain hemorrhage, etc.).

Arteriosclerosis—narrowing and hardening of the arteries due to plaque buildup of fats and cholesterol. This leads to blood clots and heart-related diseases.

Artery—a blood vessel that carries oxygen-rich blood to organs and tissues.

Arthralgia—joint pain.

Arthritis—pain and stiffness in one or more joints due to inflammation.

Articular—a word that is used in reference to a joint or multiple joints.

Atrophy—loss of or wasting away, usually in reference to muscles or organs, resulting from inactivity or cell degeneration.

Balneotherapy—treatment of a disorder by bathing. It is used widely for arthritis and neuromuscular disorders.

Bronchitis—inflammation of the bronchi in the lungs due to bacterial or viral infection. This results in shortness of breath and coughing up thick mucus.

Bulimia—an eating disorder in which an individual binge eats and then forcefully purges (throws up) often due to poor self-image.

Bursa—small, fluid-filled sacs that facilitate the movement of tendons and muscles across hard, bony surfaces.

Calluses—thick, hardened areas of skin resulting from excessive friction.

Carpal tunnel syndrome—pinching of nerves in the wrist that leads to tingling, numbness, and discomfort in the hand.

Cartilage—firm but flexible connective tissue that connects to the end of bone allowing smooth joint formation and preventing bone-on-bone friction.

Catheter—a thin tube inserted into the body and utilized in various medical situations (i.e., surgery, urination, etc.).

Cellulitis—inflammation of the cells of the skin due to a bacterial skin infection.

Chorea—a neurological disease that causes unpredictable involuntary movement of the body, normally in the face, hips, legs, and arms.

Chronic—a long-lasting, constantly reoccurring disease.

Cognitive—of or relating to the brain with respect to perspective, memory, and reasoning.

Cognitive behavioral therapy—initially used to treat depression, cognitive behavioral therapy is a form of psychological treatment that changes the way patients think to change the way they feel.

Contusion—a bruise resulting from blunt force damaging muscle and tissue.

Cortisol—a steroid hormone that is released in times of stress, resulting in the suppression of the immune system and elevated blood glucose levels.

C-reactive protein—a protein, often screened for in blood tests, that is found in the blood in response to inflammation.

Dementia—a term used to characterize a group of diseases associated with memory loss, disorientation, and mental incapacitation.

Diagnosis—through the recognition of related symptoms, the identification of a disease.

Dopamine—a neurotransmitter that regulates the brain's reward and pleasure systems.

Embryonic stem cell—stem cells that are derived from embryos that have the ability to differentiate into many types of cells.

Emphysema—a chronic disease of the lungs due to blockage of the alveoli (fluid-filled air sacs) leading to shortness of breath. Emphysema is most often caused by cigarette smoking.

Encephalitis—acute inflammation of the brain, most commonly due to a viral infection.

Enemas—a drug, liquid, or gas that is inserted into the rectum to promote defecation and clean the colon.

Enzymatic therapy—an enzyme diet treatment that utilizes herbal and animal enzymes in an attempt to restore normal human metabolic and enzymatic activity.

Epilepsy—also known as a seizure, epilepsy is a neurological disorder in which the nerve cells in the brain fire abnormally and uncontrollably.

Erythrocyte sedimentation rate—a common lab test that estimates the level of inflammation by measuring the rate that red blood cells sediment in a test tube over the period of an hour.

Fibromyalgia—a common, chronic condition of widespread pain, fatigue, and tenderness of the body.

Fibromyositis—widespread inflammation of fibrous tissue and muscle leading to pain.

Gout—a type of arthritis that leads to pain and tenderness in the joints.

Hippocampus—a section of the brain that controls mood, memory formation, and the autonomic nervous system.

Homeopathic—a type of alternative medicine, often referred to as pseudoscience because it is often not supported by credible research.

Hypersomnia—a sleep condition characterized by excessive tiredness, prolonged sleeping at night, and abnormal daytime fatigue and sleepiness.

Hypochondria—a condition in which patients obsessively worry about having a health condition where none may be present.

Hypoglycemia—lower than normal blood glucose levels.

Hypothalamus—a portion of the brain that controls homeostasis, or the body's internal balance, by releasing or inhibiting hormones that regulate sleep, appetite, heart rate, and thirst, to name a few.

Hypothyroidism—lower than normal thyroid levels in the body leading to symptoms such as fatigue, sensitivity to cold, and weight gain.

Idiopathic—a term used to describe a disease of unknown origin.

Inflammation—a localized condition in response to infection or injury where there is an accumulation of white blood cells, swelling, heat, and often pain.

Insomnia—a sleep disorder in which it is difficult to fall asleep and stay asleep.

Insulin—a hormone that regulates blood glucose levels by promoting cell uptake of blood glucose.

Interleukin-6—a group of signaling proteins that both increases inflammation during infection as well as decreases inflammation of muscle cells during exercise.

Interleukin-8—a group of signaling proteins that stimulates the immune system in response to an infection as well as promotes blood vessel formation.

Interstitial cystitis—a painful, chronic inflammation of the bladder walls.

Irritable bowel syndrome—a painful intestinal disorder that causes abdominal cramping, bloating, constipation, and diarrhea.

Leprosy—an infectious disease that causes skin lesions, nerve cell damage, and painful skin sensitivity due to a bacterial infection.

Libido—an individual's desire for sex.

Ligaments—fibrous connective tissue between bone and bone.

Lupus—a chronic inflammatory autoimmune disease where the body attacks its own cells leading to rashes, pain, fatigue, and other systems.

Lymph nodes—nodules in the body that store lymphocytes, the body's immune cells, and filters lymph fluid.

Meningiomas—usually benign (noncancerous) tumors that form along the meninges located along the brain and the spinal cord.

Meningitis—inflammation of the meninges, or protective layer, that surrounds the brain and spinal cord due to viral, bacterial, or fungal infections.

Myalgia—pain in a muscle or group of muscles.

Myasthenia—a neuromuscular disease that leads to the fatigue of voluntary muscle and muscle weakness.

Myelopathy—a neurological disorder of the spinal cord, commonly from spinal cord compression.

Myitis—muscle inflammation.

Myodysneuria—painful urination.

Myofascial—relating to fascia, or connective tissue, that surrounds the muscle.

Narcolepsy—a neurological sleep disorder that leads to daytime drowsiness and sudden onset of sleep.

Narcotics—commonly used for pain relief, narcotics are drugs that induce sleep.

Neuralgia—nerve pain.

Neurasthenia—a poorly defined condition characterized by fatigue, generalized muscle weakness, and headaches.

Neuron—also known as a nerve cell, a neuron transmits electrical and chemical signals throughout the body.

Neuropeptide Y—a protein signal that is usually released in response to low blood glucose levels to promote hunger and inhibit physical exertion.

Neurosyphilis—a condition in which syphilis bacteria infect the brain and spinal cord leading to various symptoms, including loss of motor function and mental confusion.

Neurotransmitters—chemical messengers that travel across the synapse, or space between neurons, to transfer information to other neurons.

Noggin—a protein that plays a major role in neural induction and is required for joint formation.

Nystagmus—an eye disorder that results in involuntary and unpredictable eye movements, making it difficult to see.

Pallor—a condition in which there is a lack of oxygenated blood flowing to areas of the body leading to a pale appearance, usually occurring in the face and extremities.

Palpitations—abnormal rapid beating of the heart.

Paracusis—a hearing disorder.

Parasympathetic nervous system—the part of the nervous system responsible for regulating involuntary movement and unconscious actions such as breathing, heart rate, and digestion.

Paresthesia—a sometimes painful tingling sensation that occurs when nerves are damaged or forcefully pressed.

Parkinson's disease—a chronic progressive disease of the nervous system that results in uncontrolled trembling movement.

Phakoma—a rare, small, grayish-white tumor observed in the retina in tuberous sclerosis cases.

Phthalates—A group of man-made chemicals used in plastics and solvents.

Polygenic—a phenotypic trait that derived from multiple genes.

Primary prevention—methods to prevent disease prior to onset (i.e., exercise to prevent obesity).

Psychogenic rheumatism—inflammation of joints and muscle generated by psychological issues.

Restless leg syndrome—a neurological condition characterized by a strong, unpleasant desire to move the legs.

Rheumatism—inflammation of the joints and muscles.

Rhinitis—inflammation of the mucosal lining in the nose that leads to runny and stuffy nose.

Sjögren's syndrome—an autoimmune disease that leads to dry mouth and dry eyes.

Substance P—a protein that regulates inflammation and perception of pain.

Symptoms—an objective indicator of disease, mainly characterized by health care professionals.

Temporomandibular joint syndrome—a disorder accompanied by painful sensations to the muscles and nerves of the jaw due to a damaged temporomandibular joint.

Tendons—thick, connective tissue that connects muscle to bone.

Tinnitus—a buzzing sound in the ear when there is actually no sound.

Toxemia—an accumulation of environmental toxins in the human body that leads to symptoms of fatigue, irritability, and mental confusion.

FOR FURTHER READING

Campbell D. Fibromyalgia Well-Being. Balboa Press; 2012.

Elrod JM. Reversing Fibromyalgia: The Whole-Health Approach to Overcoming Fibromyalgia Through Nutrition, Exercise, Supplements and Other Lifestyle Factors. Woodland Publishing; 2nd edition 2002.

Florence M, Marek CC. The First Year: Fibromyalgia: An Essential Guide for the Newly Diagnosed. Da Capo Press; 2003.

Fransen J, Russell IJ. The Fibromyalgia Help Book: Practical Guide to Living Better with Fibromyalgia. Smith House Press; 13th edition 1997.

Goldenberg DL. Fibromyalgia: A Leading Expert's Guide to Understanding and Getting Relief from the Pain That Won't Go Away. The Berkley Publishing Group; 2002.

Hennen W. Fibromyalgia: A Nutritional Approach. Woodland Publishing; 1999.

Liptan G. Figuring out Fibromyalgia: Current Science and the Most Effective Treatments. Visceral Books LLC; 1st edition 2011.

Mcllwain HH. The Fibromyalgia Handbook: A 7-Step Program to Halt and Even Reverse Fibromyalgia. Holt Paperbacks; 3rd edition 2003.

Murphree R. Treating and Beating Fibromyalgia and Chronic Fatigue Syndrome. Harrison & Hampton Publishing; 5th edition 2013.

Ostalecki S. Fibromyalgia: The Complete Guide from Medical Experts and Patients. Jones & Bartlett Learning; 1st edition 2007.

Rawlings D, Teitelbaum J. Foods That Fight Fibromyalgia: Nutrient-Packed Meals That Increase Energy, Ease Pain, and Move You Toward Recovery. Fair Winds Press; 2012.

Smith W, Meyler Z. Exercises for Fibromyalgia: The Complete Exercise Guide for Managing and Lessening Fibromyalgia Symptoms. Hatherleigh Press; 1st edition 2013.

Starlanyl D. The Fibromyalgia Advocate: Getting the Support You Need to Cope with Fibromyalgia and Myofascial Pain Syndrome. New Harbinger Publications, Inc.; 1st edition 1999.

Starlanyl D, Copeland ME. Fibromyalgia & Chronic Myofascial Pain: A Survival Manual. New Harbinger Publications; 2001.

Teitelbaum J. The Fatigue and Fibromyalgia Solution: The Essential Guide to Overcoming Chronic Fatigue and Fibromyalgia, Made Easy! Avery; 1st edition 2013.

Wallace DJ, Clauw DJ. Fibromyalgia & Other Central Pain Syndromes. Lippincott Williams & Wilkins; 2005.

Wallace DJ, Wallace JB. All About Fibromyalgia. Oxford University Press; 2002.

INDEX

Aaron, L., 171n9
Adams, N., 178n3
Afari, N., 171n4
Alciati, A., 173n2
Altomonte, L., 173n2
alternative therapies, 79; acupuncture, 86;
    chiropractic therapy, 84; cold therapy,
    89; heat therapy, 88; herbal options,
    80; homeopathy, 89; hydrotherapy, 88;
    positional release therapy, 84;
    transcranial magnetic stimulation, 83;
    transcutaneous electrical nerve
    stimulation, 79; trigger point therapy,
    86
Ambrus, J. Jr, 175n19
American College of Rheumatology, 51;
    ACR 1990, xiv
American Medical Association, 6
antidepressant side effects, 101; agitated
    state of mind, 101; anxiousness, 102;
    constipation or diarrhea, 102;
    headaches and migraine, 102; inability
    to sleep well, 102; loss of appetite, 102;
    repeated bouts of dizziness, 102;
    stomachaches and indigestion, 102;
    tiredness or fatigue, 102
anxiety, 183n7
Arnold, M., 167n4, 175n23, 179n8
Arioli, G., 173n2
Arnold, L. M., 178n4

assessments of FM symptoms, 60;
    language and speech, 60; memory and
    cognition, 60; muscle strength and
    restrictive movement, 60; nerves in the
    neck and head, 60; overall balance and
    posture, 60; reflexes, 60
Ashton, S., 171n9
Asukai, N., 177n4
Atzeni, F., 173n2
Aublet-Cuvellier, 177n11

Bäckman, E., 174n14
Baert, I., 177n9
Bake, B., 175n21
balance predicaments, 174n11; associated
    neck extension or rotation, 23;
    spinning rooms and, 23
Balfour, William, 3
Baldwin, D., 177n6
Barbasetti, N., 173n1, 175n24
Barjola, P., 173n6
basic self-care guidelines, 43; exercising
    guidelines, 43; reducing stress, 43;
    regulating sleep hours, 43
Bazzichi, L., 173n2
Beard, George, 4
Beena, J., 179n9
Bell, M. J., 169n20
Belcourt, M., 171n9
Bellato, E., 172n24, 173n1
Bengtsson, A., 168n2, 174n14

ABOUT THE AUTHOR

Naheed Ali, MD, PhD, began writing professionally in 2005, and he has taught at colleges where he lectured on various biomedical topics. Additional information is available online at NaheedAli.com.